Combination Drug Therapy for Hypertension

Combination Drug Therapy for Hypertension

Edited by

Lionel H. Opie, M.D, D.Phil., F.R.C.P
Professor of Medicine
Director, Medical Research Council
Ischemic Heart Disease Unit
University of Cape Town
Cape Town, South Africa

Visiting Professor
Division of Cardiovascular Medicine
Stanford University Medical Center
Stanford, California

Franz H. Messerli, M.D.
Professor of Internal Medicine
Ochsner Clinic and
Alton Ochsner Medical Foundation
New Orleans, Louisiana

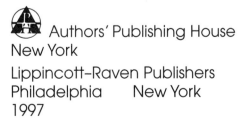 Authors' Publishing House
New York
Lippincott–Raven Publishers
Philadelphia   New York
1997

Every effort has been made to check generic and trade names, and to verify drug doses as correct according to the standards accepted at the time of publication. The ultimate responsibility lies with prescribing physicians, based on their professional experience and knowledge of the patient, to determine dosages and the best course of treatment for the patient. The reader is advised to check the product information currently provided by the manufacturer of each drug to be administered to ascertain any change in drug dosage, method of administration, or contraindications. In no case can the institutions with which the authors are affiliated or the publisher be held responsible for the views expressed in this book, which reflects the combined opinions of several authors. Please call any errors to the attention of the authors.

ISBN: 1-881063-05-4

Printed in the United States of America

CONTENTS

George L. Bakris, M.D., F.A.C.P.
Department of Preventive and Internal Medicine
Rush Presbyterian-St. Luke's Medical Center
Suite 117
1725 West Harrison Street
Chicago, Illinois 60612

Gustav G. Belz, M.D., Ph.D.
Arzt für Innere Medizin Kardiologie
Alwinenstrasse 16
D-6200 Wiesbaden
Germany

William H. Frishman, M.D.
Professor and Associate Chairman
Department of Medicine
Albert Einstein College Hospital
Montefiore Medical Center
1825 Eastchester Road
Bronx, New York 10461-2373

Ehud Grossman, M.D.
Hypertension Unit
The Chaim Sheba Medical Center
Tel-Hashomer
Israel

Lennart Hansson, M.D., Ph.D.
Clinical Hypertension Research
Department of Geriatrics
University of Uppsala
P.O. Box 609
75125 Uppsala
Sweden

Norman M. Kaplan, M.D.
Professor of Internal Medicine
Head of Hypertension Division
University of Texas Southwestern Medical Center
5233 Harry Hines Boulevard
Dallas, Texas 75235-8899

Prasad K. Kilaru, M.D.
Assistant Professor of Medicine
Division of Adult Cardiology
Cook County Hospital and
Rush Presbyterian-St. Luke's Medical Center
1835 W. Harrison Street
Chicago, Illinois 60612

Thomas F. Lüscher, M.D.
Professor and Head of Cardiology
University Hospital
CH-8091 Zurich
Switzerland

Giuseppe Mancia, M.D.
Professor of Medicine
University of Milan
Head, Division of Internal Medicine
S. Gerardo Hospital
Via Donizetti 106
20052 Milan
Italy

Franz H. Messerli, M.D.
Professor of Internal Medicine
Ochsner Clinic and
Alton Ochsner Medical Foundation
1514 Jefferson Highway
New Orleans, Louisiana 70121

Pierre Moreau
Research Fellow
Division of Cardiology
University Hospital
CH-3010 Bern
Switzerland

Lionel H. Opie, M.D., D.Phil., F.R.C.P.
Professor of Medicine
Director, Medical Research Council
Ischemic Heart Disease Unit
University of Cape Town
Cape Town
South Africa
and
Visiting Professor
Division of Cardiovascular Medicine
Stanford University Medical Center
Stanford, California

Hiroyuki Taskase
Research Fellow
Division of Cardiology
University Hospital
CH-3010 Bern
Switzerland

Michael A. Weber, M.D.
Chairman, Department of Medicine
Brookdale University Hospital and Medical Center
Professor of Medicine
State University of New York
Health Science Center
One Brookdale Plaza
Brooklyn, New York 11212-3198

Myron H. Weinberger, M.D.
Professor of Medicine
Director, Hypertension Research Center
Indiana University School of Medicine
Room 423
541 Clinical Drive
Indianapolis, Indiana 46202-5111

Matthew R. Weir, M.D.
Professor and Director
Division of Nephrology and Clinical Research Unit
Department of Medicine
Box 168
University of Maryland Medical Center
22 South Greene Street
Baltimore, Maryland 21201-1595

René R. Wenzel, M.D.
Division of Cardiology
University Hospital
CH-3010 Bern
Switzerland

When an approved treatment is considered for an unapproved indication, the physician must evaluate the safety of the medication, its value in related conditions, and the individual patient. What is asked is that he make a prudent decision based upon full knowledge of the available evidence.

—Judge's instruction to jury

Hypertension remains one of the major causes of cardiovascular mortality, which in turn is the most readily identifiable cause of death in western countries. In emerging economies, including countries such as South Africa, the pattern of death from hypertension shifts from a predominantly cardiovascular mechanism, as found in the United States, to stroke, but the importance of hypertension as a major cause of death remains. Furthermore, hypertension is recognized as a foremost cause of morbidity, especially in the increasingly important and numerous elderly population.

Although there are many recommendations made for the initial drug treatment of hypertension according to the principle of monotherapy, the reality is that many (if not most) patients either need or would benefit from combination drug treatment. The fifth report of the Joint National Committee on Detection, Evaluation and Treatment of High Blood Pressure states that combining antihypertensive drugs with different modes of action will often allow smaller doses to be used to achieve control of blood pressure, thereby minimizing the potential for dose-dependent side effects. Yet despite the common use of combination therapy, there are no guidelines or books solely devoted to such combination therapy.

Our aim in this book is to guide the physician in the choice of drugs for combination therapy. The three major principles of combination therapy will be considered. First, *there is additive antihypertensive potency.* Because it still is not clear why some groups of patients respond better to one type of drug than another, the combination of two different drugs acting by two different mechanisms is more likely to reduce blood pressure in any given patient. Second, *side effects are often less.* The added antihypertensive effects of two different types of drugs allow for a lower dose of each to be used to achieve the same degree of blood pressure lowering. Because side effects of the various drugs are often dose related, it further follows that combination therapy is in general associated with fewer adverse side effects. Third, *complementary hemodynamic, neurohumoral, and metabolic mechanisms of the two types of drugs may achieve synergistic effects.* For example, low doses of a diuretic and a beta-blocker, neither capable of effectively reducing blood pressure on their own, are licensed for this purpose. Probably, the diuretic has its hypotensive effect limited by reactive release of renin from the kidneys, and this adverse response may be counterbalanced by the capacity of a beta-blockade to lessen renal release of renin. Diuretic-induced hypokalemia can be blunted by adding a beta-blocker or an angiotensin-converting enzyme (ACE) inhibitor. Likewise, there are good arguments given in this book for combining angiotensin II receptor blockers with diuretics or even with ACE inhibitors, and for combination therapy with beta-blockers and calcium antagonists. Likewise there are increasing arguments for combining ACE inhibitors and calcium antagonists.

Because there are at least five major antihypertensive mechanisms and numerous drugs in each category, the possible number of combinations of such drugs is endless. We have, therefore, selected and described those drug combinations that are of specific theoretical interest or are especially well used. Then we have selected crucial issues to discuss, such as the capacity of combination therapy to control stroke and renal disease, and risk factors for coronary atherosclerosis. Finally, long-term safety is considered because of increasing concern that drugs should not only have short-term benefits, but should prolong life and decrease morbidity.

We have been greatly aided in these ambitious tasks by the chapter authors, who are highly respected in the world of hypertension. We optimistically predict that this book will fill an important need and have a major impact.

L.H. Opie
F.H. Messerli

CHAPTER 1

Principles of Combination Therapy for Hypertension

Lionel H. Opie

The major aim in the therapy of hypertension remains reduction of blood pressure. The simplest hypothesis for the benefits of treatment of hypertension is that blood pressure lowering will lessen end organ damage. Provided that blood pressure reduction is obtained throughout 24 hours and excess hypotension is avoided, better blood pressure control should give better results. This hypothesis is being tested in the Hypertension Optimal Treatment (HOT) trial in which the initial drug is the calcium antagonist felodipine, with scope for combination treatment by an angiotensin–converting enzyme (ACE) inhibitor or a beta-blocker (1). The aim is to establish which diastolic blood pressure level is optimal to avoid complications (90, 85, or 80 mmHg). This trial will reveal both the ideal diastolic blood pressure for which to aim during antihypertensive therapy and whether combination drug therapy is effective in reaching that ideal.

Thus, till disproved, blood pressure reduction is the crucial and overriding aim. Yet the various guidelines issued by the many guiding bodies often suggest first-line therapy by low-dose diuretics. For example, the Canadian Hypertension Society recommends an initial therapy of hydrochlorothiazide 25 mg (2). The Fifth Joint National Committee (JNC-V) gives preference to diuretics or beta-blockers and suggests a dose of hydrochlorothiazide 12.5 to 50 mg daily (3). Using the example of the diuretics, this chapter will argue that adequate blood pressure reduction may not be achievable by diuretic monotherapy without risk of metabolic side effects, whereas combination therapy of low-dose diuretics and another agent such as a beta-blocker or an ACE inhibitor would be preferable. Examples of metabolically advantageous combinations are that of a calcium antagonist with a beta-blocker or with an ACE inhibitor. Other projected effects of combination therapy are shown in Table 1-1.

TABLE 1-1. SUMMARY OF EFFECTS OF COMBINATION ANTIHYPERTENSIVE THERAPY

Drug Class	BP Fall	Meta-bolic	Blood Lipids	Stroke Effect	CHD Effect	LVH Effect	Renal Effect	Safety	Outcome
D	+, slow	Neg	Neg	Yes	Fair	?	GFR↓	Poor*	Good
βB	+	?OK	Neg	Yes	No	+	?	Poor**	Mixed
D + βB	++	Neg‡	Neg	Yes‡	No‡	?+	?	Fair	Good‡
D, ACE	++	Neutral	Neutral	?	?	?+	? Good	?Good	?Good
C, βB	++	Neutral	Neutral	?	?	?++	?	?Fair	?Good
C, ACE	++	Neutral†	Neutral	?	?	?+++	Yes†	?Good	?Good
α com	++	Neutral	Pos	?	? Pos	?+	?	?Good	?Good

+ = positive effect; ++ = more positive effect; +++ = marked positive effect; BP = blood pressure; CHD = coronary heart disease; LVH = left ventricular hypertrophy; D = diuretic; βB = beta-blocker; ACE = angiotensin-converting enzyme inhibitor; C = calcium channel antagonist; α com = alpha-blocker combinations; Neg = negative data (i.e., adverse effects on blood lipid profile); Pos = positive data; GFR = glomerular filtration rate.
* High dose: risk of sudden death, diabetes, gout, renal cancer(4).
** MRC trial in elderly; Weinmann, et al. (4); Hoes et al. (5); Siscovick et al.(6).
†= Schneider et al. (7).
‡= Data from the Swedish Trial in Old Patients with Hypertension (STOP-Hypertension); see Chapter 13.

WHY MONOTHERAPY MAY FAIL: THE 40-YEAR-OLD SAGA OF DIURETICS

The two major reasons why monotherapy may fail are, first, the dose of the drug may be too low and, second, the mechanism whereby the drug acts is unlikely to work in the patient under consideration. The question of drug dose may seem to be of lesser importance when considering that diuretics, among the first class of drugs introduced, are still considered among the best first-line choices for monotherapy. Soon after the introduction of these drugs it became apparent that the dose response to these drugs was flat (8). Yet even today, after about 40 years of experience, arguments still rage about the optimal dose of diuretic drugs. The current trend is to recommend low doses, with the aim of avoiding or minimizing metabolic side effects while hopefully retaining hypotensive efficacy (on the principle of "having your cake and eating it"). How valid are these expectations?

Do Trial Data Really Show That Low-Dose Diuretics Are Adequately Antihypertensive?

The short answer is "no" except in the elderly (9) and in those who have very mild hypertension (10). Several trials have shown that there *is* a dose-response antihypertensive effect with diuretics, at least in the dose range of 12.5 to 50 mg hydrochlorothiazide. Doses at the bottom end of the range are unlikely to work as monotherapy. Taking two recent examples, in the Pollare study (11), which compared the metabolic effects of equieffective doses of an ACE inhibitor and a diuretic, Pollare and colleagues found that the average dose of hydrochlorothiazide required was close to 50 mg, well above the "desired" level of 25 mg or less. In the Veterans Administration (VA) study (12), an average dose of about 40 mg hydrochlorothiazide was needed to achieve blood pressure reduction, which on the whole was not as good as that found by the calcium antagonist diltiazem. It is true that in the Treatment of Mild Hypertension (TOMH) study over 4 years, low-dose chlorthalidone (15 mg daily) was considered effective, yet there are two important reservations. First, the subjects were minimally hypertensive with entry blood pressure levels close to 140/90 mmHg and, second, they were all on a salt-restricted, weight-reducing diet (10). It is also true that low-dose chlorthalidone (15 mg daily) given to elderly subjects with systolic hypertension reduced hard end points such as stroke and cardiac disease, as well as overall mortality (9). Yet, again, there are two major reservations. First, it is not known what percentage of patients required combination therapy with the second drug of choice, a beta-blocker. Second, the elderly patients under consideration were, in general, a group in whom salt sensitivity is common, so that a relatively good response to a low-dose diuretic can logically be expected. For example, in the VA study (12), the response to diuretic monotherapy was better in those 60 years old and older, rather than in the younger patients. Thus, the hard evidence that low-dose diuretics would generally be effective or protective in pre-elderly hypertensive patients remains to be gathered.

Low Diuretic Doses and Metabolic Safety

The major argument for the desirability of low-dose diuretic therapy rests on the side effect profiles. Metabolically, the low doses are less prone to cause hypokalemia, glucose intolerance, and hyperlipidemia (13, 14). Therapeutically effective doses of diuretics, such as hydrochlorothiazide doses of about 40 mg daily, increase blood glucose values (12) and, by inference, promote insulin resistance. Whether the lipid effects of even low-dose diuretics can be ignored is a matter of dispute. In a preliminary report (15), blood cholesterol changes found in over 1,000 hypertensives given hydrochlorothiazide for 1 to 2 years were no different from those in groups treated by an ACE inhibitor, an alpha-blocker, or a calcium antagonist. The diuretic dose was not stated, but judging from a parallel publication (12), could have been 40 mg hydrochlorothiazide. A low dose of chlorthalidone, 15 mg daily, increased the blood cholesterol level at 1 year but not at 4 years (10).

Much might depend on the preexisting metabolic characteristics of the patient under consideration. For example, in exercising nonobese individuals with normal or even supernormal glucose tolerance, and with a good blood lipid profile, a diuretic even in medium doses might not cause much concern. On the other hand, few would be happy at giving a diuretic, except in really low doses, to patients who already have impaired glucose tolerance, as in mature onset type 2 diabetes. Diuretic-linked increases in mortality may occur, especially in diabetics (16). Another population prone to metabolic mishaps with diuretic therapy may be middle-age black females in whom thiazide, 25 to 50 mg daily over 5 years, increased blood glucose and cholesterol, according to a preliminary report (17).

High-Dose Diuretics and Potentially Lethal Cardiac Complications

In mild to moderate hypertension, the degree of hypokalemia induced by low-dose thiazide seldom matters (18). On the other hand, it cannot be disputed that diuretic therapy with doses such as 50 mg hydrochlorothiazide, often used and declared the top dose by JNC-V, may predispose to hypokalemia (12) with risk of arrhythmias such as torsades de pointes, a potentially fatal arrhythmia (19). Furthermore, a case control study (Figure 1-1) suggests that 50 mg hydrochlorothiazide daily, given for hypertension, is associated with about three times an increased risk of primary cardiac arrest than the same drug in a lower dose of 25 mg daily and combined with a potassium-sparing diuretic (6). High-dose thiazide, 100 mg per day without potassium-sparing therapy, has a risk that is *eight times* higher (6). In another study, either diuretic or β-blocker therapy for hypertension increased the risk of sudden cardiac death by about 1.7 times (5), when compared with the reference group primarily treated by potassium-sparing diuretics. The harmful diuretic doses are not stated but judging from the years of data collection (1988–1990), the doses could well have been high. While such case control studies have severe inherent limitations, they can be

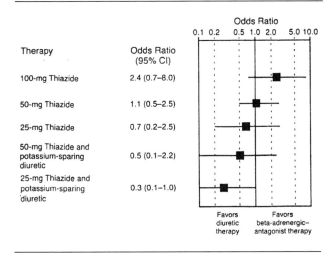

Figure 1-1. Role of cardiac arrest in patients with hypertension treated by thiazide diuretics with or without a potassium-sparing diuretic. Note increased risk with (a) high-dose thiazide; (b) β-blocker therapy. From Siscovick et al. (1994) with permission (6).

useful in the formulation of hypotheses. Further evidence comes from the large MRC study which compared high dose bendrofluazide with propranolol in middle-aged men; the incidence of sudden death was more than twice as high in the diuretic group (p=0.01)(20). Because hypokalemia predisposes to serious ventricular arrhythmias, and because high diuretic doses predispose to hypokalemia, such severe cardiac complications are not unexpected.

Thus the cardiovascular safety data strongly favor low-dose diuretics and the combination therapy by a thiazide type diuretic with a potassium-sparing agent such as amiloride or triamterene. The safety and efficacy of such combinations have already been shown in two large trials on elderly hypertensive patients, the EWPHE study (21) and the MRC study on the elderly (22). Similar arguments would favor the combination of thiazide with an ACE inhibitor.

Other Adverse Effects of Diuretics

In addition to the cardiovascular risk, diuretics have the clinically well-known propensity to provoke, in the susceptible, diabetes mellitus and gout. For example, over 30 years ago Cranston and associates warned: "Clearly diabetes induced by diuretics cannot be dismissed as a trivial side-effect"(8, p. 970). A serious risk that is often ignored is the increased incidence of renal carcinoma with chronic diuretic use, with chronic hypokalemia as a possible mechanism (4).

Diuretic Response: The Importance of Age and Ethnicity

The VA study (12) showed that diuretic monotherapy, even at a mean thiazide dose of about 40 mg daily, left younger (age less than 60) white males virtually untouched, whereas there was an excellent response in elderly black males (9). These responses could perhaps have been predicted because diuretic monotherapy should theoretically work best in those with a preexisting low renin status, as in the elderly or in black subjects. The logic would be that diuretics invoke a renin-angiotensin response that is counterregulatory. Hypothetically, starting with a low renin status allows for more latitude for this adverse effect than does an initial high renin status.

Diuretic Data: What Do They All Add Up To?

Thus there is good evidence favoring the view that the lower the dose of diuretic, the safer for the patient, but the less chance diuretic monotherapy is effectively antihypertensive. In addition, certain population groups such as younger white patients might be particularly resistant to diuretics, while others such as the elderly and black patients might be more susceptible to such therapy. But taking the population as a whole, it can safely be prophesied that low-dose diuretic therapy by itself is often likely to be inadequately hypotensive. This conclusion does not exclude the possibility that low-dose diuretic therapy might be still be highly cost-effective when compared with more expensive treatment, but it does emphasize that in reality combination therapy is often going to be required.

REASONS FOR THE ADDITIVE ANTIHYPERTENSIVE POTENCY OF COMBINATION THERAPY

1. The net is cast wider. If different population groups might respond differently to different groups of antihypertensive therapy, then a combination of agents acting together would have a greater statistical chance of success. Ideally of course, we would know which population groups would respond best to which drugs and then start with the appropriate monotherapy. This requirement would call for many more studies than that of the VA(12), which was confined to male veterans. In particular, females, obese subjects, and noninsulin-dependent diabetics would all need a similar comparison of six different groups of drugs. And even more ideally, those failing monotherapy would then go on to drug combinations. In the absence of such detailed knowledge, all that can be said with certainty is that combination therapy is more likely to decrease the blood pressure of more patients by a greater amount than monotherapy.

2. Side effects are fewer. The net can catch more fish without the fish noticing the net. Because many and probably most side effects are dose related, and because side effects differ between the drug groups, it follows that when an equal antihypertensive effect is obtained by a combination of two drugs from two different groups, the side effect profile can be expected to be lower. This principle should apply to subjective as well as to objective side effects, but is not relevant to idiosyncratic events such as angioedema with the ACE inhibitors. Some examples are as follows. Metabolic side effects of diuretics can be diminished by a combination of low-dose diuretics with an ACE inhibitor (Chapter 4) or with a beta-blocker (e.g., bisoprolol with a very low dose of thiazide, 6.25 mg daily, as discussed in Chapter 3). Attractive, too, are the combinations of drug groups that in themselves have no metabolic side effects, such as the ACE inhibitors and the calcium antagonists, or drug groups with metabolic benefit, such as the alpha-blockers, with others that might have converse effects, such as the beta-blockers.

3. *The drugs have additive pharmacological properties. The net is stronger.* Different groups of drugs have varying hemodynamic features that could be additive. For example, (1) diuretics decrease the circulating blood volume; (2) beta-blockers decrease the heart rate and cardiac output while tending to increase the peripheral vascular resistance; (3) vasodilators, including the ACE inhibitors, calcium antagonists, and alpha-blockers all decrease the peripheral vascular resistance; and (4) centrally active agents decrease the sympathetic outflow. Different vasodilators act on different sites on the cell membrane, the calcium antagonists on the calcium channel, the ACE inhibitors on the angiotensin receptor by decreasing the formation of angiotensin II, the angiotensin receptor blockers by directly competing with angiotensin for the level of the receptor, and the alpha-blockers at the $alpha_1$-adrenergic receptor. Therefore, different vasodilators should be additive in their effects.

4. *Different drug groups have complementary properties, thereby neutralizing the adverse effects of the individual components. The net catches more fish than expected.* Diuretics, stimulating the renin-angiotensin system, are ideally combined with ACE inhibitors and with angiotensin receptor blockers. Alternately, diuretics may be combined with beta-blockers, which inhibit the release rather than the effects of renin. Calcium antagonists of the nifedipine group (the dihydropyridines) increase circulating catecholamines and tend to activate the renin-angiotensin system. Thus such drugs may be logically combined with ACE inhibitors or beta-blockers, both combinations being commercially available. Calcium antagonists of the verapamil group tend to decrease circulating catecholamines so that combination with a beta-blockade is not logical. Rather, combination with another vasodilator, such as an ACE inhibitor, becomes attractive. Centrally active agents, being hemodynamically neutral, can be combined with all the other groups of agents, provided that the central effects can be tolerated.

5. *Different drugs can have complementary actions on specific end organs. The net can catch more fish of a certain species.* For example, in the case of renal circulation, the calcium antagonists decrease afferent arteriolar tone, whereas the ACE inhibitors chiefly act on the efferent arteriole. Thus the intraglomerular pressure should be better reduced by the combination of these drugs, which may explain the superior reduction of diabetic microalbuminuria by the combination of verapamil and ACE inhibitor (23). Likewise it is possible to predict that this combination is more likely to provide postinfarct protection than either alone, because verapamil is anti-ischemic but tends to cause heart failure, whereas the

ACE inhibitor specifically decreases left ventricular (LV) size but is only indirectly anti-ischemic.

    6. But, more is not always better. The fish will escape if many broken nets are used. The major argument against combination therapy is that any increase in the number of tablets that must be taken each day leads to a loss of compliance. This objection can be overcome by the use of fixed-combination tablets. Some of the older combinations contain too high a dose of diuretic. Compliance should be very carefully checked before any more tablets are introduced. A possible danger of combination therapy is excess hypotension, especially if a combination is started at too-high doses of the component drugs.

CRUCIAL ARGUMENTS FOR COMBINATION THERAPY

The two strongest arguments for combination therapy remain as follows. First, combination therapy gives additive or synergistic antihypertensive effects. *Complementary hemodynamic mechanisms* of the two types of drugs may achieve synergistic effects with a greater-than-expected reduction in blood pressure. For example, low doses of a diuretic and a beta-blocker, neither capable of reducing blood pressure on their own, are licensed for this purpose. Probably the diuretic has its hypotensive effect limited by reactive release of renin from the kidneys and this adverse response may be counterbalanced by the capacity of a beta-blockade to lessen renal release of renin. Second, *adverse counterregulatory mechanisms may be neutralized* by different categories of drugs. For example, peripheral vasodilation, the major mechanism by which the calcium antagonists work, invokes a counter-regulation involving adrenergic and renin-angiotensin acti-

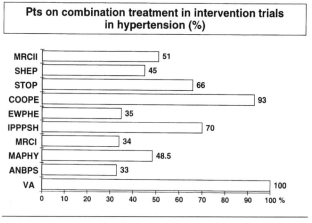

Figure 1-2. Frequency of combination antihypertensive therapy in various major trials. Note the high percentage of patients eventually treated by combination therapy despite the intent to treat by monotherapy. Courtesy of Professor G. Mancia.

vation that could be lessened by the simultaneous use of a beta-blocking drug or of an ACE inhibitor.

It must nonetheless be conceded that outcome trials with combination therapy are strictly lacking, although combination therapy has in reality been used in most existing trials (Figure 1-2). For example, in the important Swedish Trial in Old Patients (STOP) study (24), in which two-thirds of the elderly patients received combined beta-blocker plus diuretic therapy, marked reduction in stroke and total mortality was noted.

Conclusions

There are strong theoretical reasons to suppose that combination drug therapy might be better than monotherapy. If it is assumed that the efficacy of antihypertensive therapy is directly related to the degree of blood pressure reduction, then it is self-evident that different mechanisms will cast the net of therapy wider and at the cost of fewer side effects for the same degree of blood pressure lowering, because side effects differ according to the drug group chosen and are usually dose dependent. In addition, some drug combinations benefit from complementary mechanisms of action— for example, the combination of an ACE inhibitor and a diuretic, or a calcium antagonist and an ACE inhibitor.

References

1. Hansson L, Zanchetti A, The Hot Study Group. The hypertension optimal treatment (HOT) study: patient characteristics: randomization, risk profiles, and early blood pressure results. *Blood Press* 1994; 3:322–327.

2. Ogilvie RI, Burgess ED, Cusson RJ, et al. Report of the Canadian Hypertension Society Consensus Conference: 3. Pharmacologic treatment of essential hypertension. *Can Med Assoc J* 1993; 149:575–584.

3. JNC V. Joint National Committee on Detection Evaluation and Treatment of High Blood Pressure. The Fifth Report of the Joint National Committee on Detection, Evaluation and Treatment of High Blood Pressure (JNC V). *Arch Intern Med* 1993; 153:154–183.

4. Weinmann S, Glass AG, Weiss NS, et al. Use of diuretics and other antihypertensive medications in relation to the risk of renal cell cancer. *Am J Epidemiol* 1994; 140:792–804.

5. Hoes AW, Grobbee DE, Lubsen J, et al. Diuretics, β-blockers, and the risk for sudden cardiac death in hypertensive patients. *Ann Intern Med* 1995; 123:481–487.

6. Siscovick DS, Raghunathun TE, Psaty BM. Diuretic therapy for hypertension and the risk of primary cardiac arrest. *N Engl J Med* 1994; 330:1852–1857.

7. Schneider M, Lerch M, Papiri M, et al. Metabolic neutrality of combined verapramil-trandolapril treatment in contrast to beta-blocker-low-dose chlortalidone treatment in hypertensive type 2 diabetes. *J Hypertens* 1996; 14:669–677.

8. Cranston WI, Juel-Jensen BE, Semmence AM, et al. Effects of oral diuretics on raised arterial pressure. *Lancet* 1963; 2:966–969.

9. SHEP Cooperative Research Group. Prevention of stroke by antihypertensive drug treatment in older persons with isolated systolic hypertension. Final results of the systolic hypertension in the elderly program (SHEP). *JAMA* 1991; 265:3255–3264.

10. Neaton JD, Grimm RH, et al. Treatment of mild hypertension study (TOMH). Final results. *JAMA* 1993; 270:713–724.

11. Pollare T, Lithell H, Berne C. A comparison of the effects of hydrochlorothiazide and captopril on glucose and lipid metabolism in patients with hypertension. *N Engl J Med* 1989; 321:868–873.

12. Materson BJ, Reda DJ, Cushman WC, et al. Single-drug therapy for hypertension in men. A comparison of six antihypertensive agents with placebo. *N Engl J Med* 1993; 328:914–921.

13. Carlsen JE, Kober L, Torp-Pedersen C, Johansen P. Relation between dose of bendofluazide, antihypertensive effect, and adverse biochemical effects. *Br Med J* 1990; 300:975–978.

14. Jounela AJ, Lilja M, Lumme J, et al. Relation between low dose of hydrochlorothiazide, antihypertensive effect and adverse effects. *Blood Press* 1994; 3:231–235.

15. Cushman WC, Nunn SL, Lakshman MR, et al. Monotherapy of hypertension: effects of six classes of drugs and placebo on plasma lipids [abstract]. *Am J Hypertens* 1993; 6:9A.

16. Warram JH, Laffel LMB, Valsania P, et al. Excess mortality associated with diuretic therapy in diabetes mellitus. *Arch Intern Med* 1991; 151:1350–1356.

17. Elliot WJ. Glucose and cholesterol elevations from diuretic therapy: intention to treat vs actual on-therapy experience [abstract]. *Am J Hypertens* 1993; 6:9A.

18. McInnes GT, Yeo WW, Ramsay LE, Moser M. Cardiotoxicity and diuretics: much speculation—little substance. *J Hypertens* 1992; 10:317–335.

19. Parmley WW, Nesto RW, Singh BN, et al. Attenuation of the circadian patterns of myocardial ischemia with nifedipine GITS in patients with chronic stable angina. *J Am Coll Cardiol* 1992; 19:1380–1389.

20. Medical Research Council Working Party on Mild Hypertension. Coronary heart disease in the Medical Research Council trial of treatment of mild hypertension. *Br Heart J* 1988; 59:364–378.

21. Vanhees L, Aubert A, Fagard R, et al. Influence of β_1 versus β_2 adrenoreceptor blockade on left ventricular function in humans. *J Cardiovasc Pharmacol* 1986; 8:1086–1091.

22. Medical Research Council trial of treatment of hypertension in older adults: principal results. *BMJ* 1992; 304:405–412.

23. Fioretto P, Frigato F, Velussi M, et al. Effects of angiotensin converting enzyme inhibitors and calcium antagonists on atrial natriuretic peptide release and action and on albumin excretion rate in hypertensive insulin-dependent diabetic patients. *Am J Hypertens* 1992; 5:837–846.

24. Dahlöf B, Lindholm LH, et al. Morbidity and mortality in the Swedish Trial in Old Patients with hypertension (STOP-hypertension). *Lancet* 1991; 338:1281–1285.

Ambulatory Blood Pressure Monitoring for Antihypertensive Drug Studies and Combination Treatment

Giuseppe Mancia

Ambulatory blood pressure monitoring has become a customary means to determine the efficacy of antihypertensive treatment (1, 2) and a large number of studies is now available on the blood pressure-lowering effect of nonpharmacological interventions, monotherapies with different drugs, and combined administration of two or more drugs. This chapter will review the advantages of the ambulatory blood pressure approach vis-à-vis traditional blood pressure measurements for antihypertensive drug studies. It will then focus on recent evidence by ambulatory blood pressure monitoring on the antihypertensive efficacy of a relatively new combination treatment (i.e., that between an ACE inhibitor and a calcium antagonist).

THE ADVANTAGES

While clinic blood pressure is collected in an "artificial" setting, ambulatory blood pressure monitoring provides values that are close to daily life. This approach can therefore establish whether the antihypertensive effect of a given treatment does not just appear in a standardized environment, but breaks through all conditions and stimuli that may markedly affect blood pressure values per se.

This obvious advantage, however, is accompanied by other advantages that may be no less important. Studies in which ambulatory blood pressure was measured continually before, during, and after the visit of a doctor in charge of measuring blood pressure have shown that this event elicits an alerting reaction and an increase in blood pressure that is strikingly different between subjects (Figure 2-1)(3, 4). This means that clinic blood pressure measurements are affected by a variable "white-coat" effect and thus by a variable overestimation of the patients' "true" blood pressure. This can be avoided by ambulatory blood pressure monitoring, because

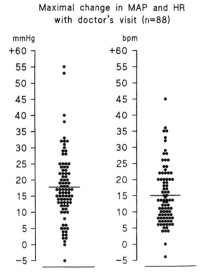

Figure 2-1. Change in systolic and diastolic blood pressure in 88 hypertensive subjects induced by a doctor's visit in whom blood pressure was measured intra-arterially before, during, and after the visit of an unfamiliar doctor in charge of measuring patients' blood pressure. Points refer to individual subjects. MAP, mean arterial pressure; HR, heart rate. (From Mancia and colleagues [3], with permission.)

the automatic blood pressure readings provided by this procedure do not modify intra-arterial blood pressure, as shown by a study in which ambulatory blood pressure was monitored in one arm and intra-arterial blood pressure in the contralateral arm in order to identify on the intra-arterial tracing the exact time at which automatic blood pressure readings were obtained (Figure 2-2) (5). This is even more important than it can *prima facie* appear, because there is now evidence that, although unchanged on a short-term basis (6), the white-coat effect may undergo an attenuation with time, leading to an overestimation of the real efficacy of antihypertensive treatment when clinic blood pressure is employed (Figure 2-3) (7)—namely, to ascribe to antihypertensive treatment an effect that is in part due to a reduced blood pressure response to clinic blood pressure measurements.

Other features of ambulatory blood pressure, however, command this approach as a highly suitable one for antihypertensive treatment studies. For example, while clinic blood pressure is variably modified by placebo, 24-hour average (as well as average day and night-time) blood pressure is largely devoid of this effect, at least when placebo is administered over a few-month period (i.e., for the time over which placebo administration is ethically acceptable) (Figure 2-4)(8–10). This means that when the efficacy of antihypertensive treatment is assessed by 24-hour, day, or nighttime average blood pressures, a placebo group (parallel study design) or phase (crossover study design) can be avoided, with a reduction in the study size, complexity, and cost. Furthermore, compared to clinical blood pressure, 24-

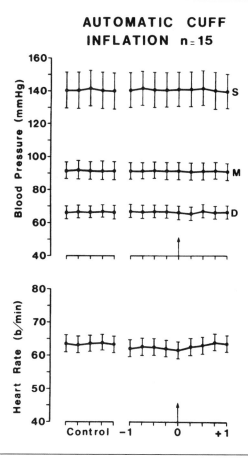

Figure 2-2. Intra-arterial blood pressure values before, during, and after cuff inflations provided by an ambulatory blood pressure monitoring device placed in the contralateral arm. Values occurring at each inflation were averaged (± standard error). The time of inflation is indicated by the arrow. S = systolic; M = mean; D = diastolic blood pressure. (From Parati and colleagues [5], with permission.)

hour average blood pressure shows a much greater reproducibility. This can be seen in Figure 2-5 in which reproducibility was measured by the Bland-Altman approach (i.e., by calculating the inverse of the standard deviation of the mean difference between two blood pressure measurements taken several weeks apart) (11). It is clear that the reproducibility of 24-hour average systolic or diastolic blood pressure increased progressively with the number of values included in the calculation of the average, reaching a plateau at which it was about three times the reproducibility of clinical blood pressure. As emphasized by Conway and Coats (12), this feature (which is shared by automatic and intra-arterial 24-hour blood pressure monitoring) implies that the number of subjects to be included in antihypertensive drug studies can be considerably reduced without any loss in the statistical power to detect a difference in the blood pressure effect. This is because by accounting for the size of unexplained and uncontrolled blood pressure variability (the back-

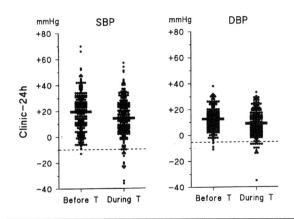

Figure 2-3. *Differences between clinic and 24-hour average blood pressure before treatment and after several weeks of treatment with different antihypertensive drugs. Points refer to individual patients. Horizontal bars represent average values. The clinic daytime blood pressure difference was taken as a surrogate measure of the white-coat effect. SBP = systolic blood pressure; DBP = diastolic blood pressure. (From Parati and colleagues [7], with permission.)*

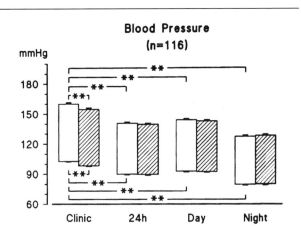

Figure 2-4. *Systolic and diastolic blood pressure before and after several weeks of placebo administration. Data are shown as mean ± standard error from 116 hypertensive patients and refer to clinic, 24-hour average, daytime average, and nighttime average blood pressure. (From Mancia and colleagues [8], with permission.)*

ground blood pressure "noise"), blood pressure reproducibility represents an important component in the calculation of the statistical power of such studies.

Several other considerations on the advantages of ambulatory blood pressure monitoring for antihypertensive drug studies should be made. First, by use of ambulatory blood pressure one can obtain information on blood pressure variability, which can be a determinant of the target organ damage related to hypertension (13–15). Second, the effect of antihypertensive treatment on night-time blood

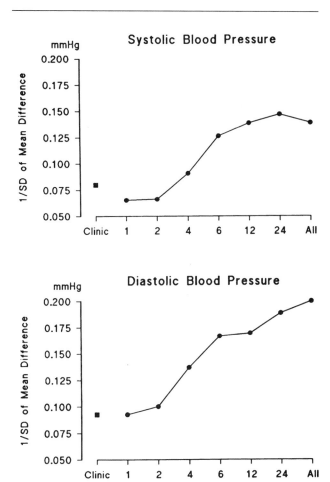

Figure 2-5. Reproducibility of clinic (square) and 24-hour average systolic and diastolic blood pressure (circle). Data were collected at month intervals. Twenty-four-hour average blood pressures were calculated by including a progressively greater number of ambulatory values. Ambulatory blood pressure was obtained by an automatic device. Reproducibility is expressed as the inverse of the standard deviation of the mean differences between the values obtained at the month interval. ABPM = ambulatory blood pressure measurement. (From Trazzi and associates [11], with permission.)

pressure can be assessed, which may be important for those who believe that (a) a high night-time blood pressure represents a specific risk (16, 17) and (b) at least in some subjects the opposite may be true (i.e., that a low night-time blood pressure may lead to vital organ underperfusion and thus that a night-time blood pressure reduction by treatment should be avoided) (18). Third, ambulatory blood pressure monitoring can identify orthostatic and other hypotensive episodes associated with treatment, which may be particularly important in elderly hypertensives and in hypertensives under treatment with multiple and/or high doses of antihypertensive drugs.

LIMITATIONS

The advantages of ambulatory blood pressure monitoring outlined earlier should not lead us to forget that this approach also has limitations. Some limitations are of a general nature and focus on the cost and time consumption inherent to this approach. Other limitations are technical and concern the fact that some devices provide blood pressure readings that have a limited accuracy, and even devices that perform very well at rest (19) lose some of their accuracy when used in ambulatory conditions (20).

There are, however, limitations that are more specific to antihypertensive drug studies. For example, as shown in Figure 2-6, ambulatory blood pressure monitorings performed before and during placebo suggest that there is a small placebo effect in the first few hours after the monitoring is started (8), although the occurrence of a similar phenomenon when a second ambulatory blood pressure monitoring is performed in absence of placebo and the lower blood pressure values observed at a time corresponding to the initial one during a second consecutive monitoring period (Figure 2-7) (21) indicate that rather than being due to placebo, the small blood pressure reduction is due to an attenuation of a startling reaction to the application of the monitoring device. This small reduction may be responsible for an error when the trough-to-peak ratio of the antihyper-

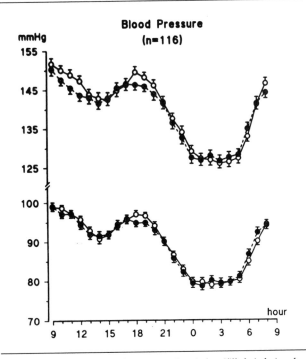

Figure 2-6. Ambulatory blood pressure values before (filled circles) and during (open circles) placebo in the same subjects of Figure 2-4. Systolic blood pressure is represented by the upper lines; diastolic blood pressure is represented by the bottom lines. Data are shown as hourly mean (± standard error) values. (From Mancia and colleagues [8], with permission.)

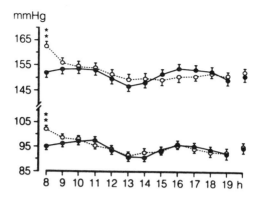

Figure 2-7. Ambulatory systolic (upper line) and diastolic (bottom line) blood pressure in hypertensive patients. Data are shown as hourly values (± standard error) for the first 12-hour and the last 12-hour period of a consecutive 36-hour ambulatory monitoring period (filled and open circles, respectively). Blood pressure was lower in the final 12 hours as compared to the initial 12-hour period. (From Zanchetti and colleagues [21], with permission.)

tensive effect is calculated based on ambulatory blood pressure data. The error consists of an overestimation of the peak blood pressure fall and thus of an underestimation of the trough-to-peak ratio that, given the small figures from which this ratio is often derived, amounts to 10% to 20%.

Furthermore, at variance from 24-hour average blood pressure, hourly blood pressure values have a variable and limited reproducibility (Figure 2-8) (22), which means that a larger number of subjects must be included in a hypertensive drug study whenever the antihypertensive effect needs to be determined with adequate statistical power throughout the 24 hours. Unfortunately, little increase in reproducibility can be obtained by increasing the number of blood pressure measurements performed within the hour, because a limited and variable hourly blood pressure reproducibility characterizes not only automatic blood pressure monitoring (two to six measurements per hour), but also intra-arterial blood pressure monitoring (about 4,000 measurements per hour) (see Figure 2-8) (22). A limited success can also be expected from behavioral standardization between different ambulatory blood pressure monitorings, because in our subjects hourly blood pressure reproducibility was limited not only during the day, but also during the night when subjects were asleep (Figure 2-9) (22). It may be possible, however, to improve reproducibility by increasing to 2 to 3 hours or 4 hours the time window over which data are averaged (23, 24), at the loss, however, of a detailed 24-hour blood pressure profile.

Finally, it should be emphasized that some of the "advantages" of ambulatory blood pressure monitoring for antihypertensive drug studies simply derive from the larger number of blood pressure values provided by this approach. This is exemplified in Figure 2-10, which shows that by increasing the number of blood pressure measurements performed in the clinic environment, blood pressure reproducibility can be

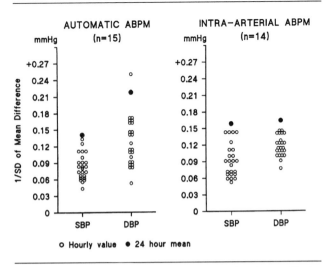

Figure 2-8. Reproducibility of 24-hour average and hourly mean blood pressure values. Reproducibility is shown as indicated in Figure 2-5. Data were obtained by automatic and intra-arterial monitoring. ABPM = ambulatory blood pressure monitoring; SBP = systolic blood pressure; DBP = diastolic blood pressure. (From Mancia and colleagues [22], with permission.)

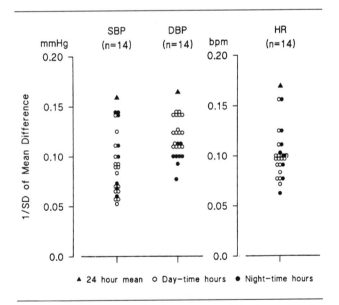

Figure 2-9. Reproducibility of 24-hour average and hourly mean blood pressure values in the subjects of Figure 2-8. Hours are indicated differently for daytime and nighttime. SBP = systolic blood pressure; DBP = diastolic blood pressure; HR = heart rate. (From Mancia and colleagues [22], with permission.)

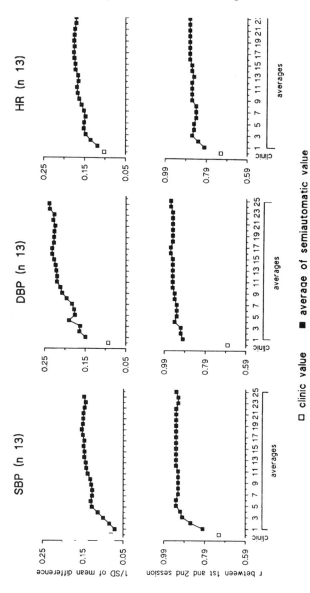

Figure 2-10. Increase in reproducibility with the increasing number of blood pressure measurements obtained in the clinic environment at one-month intervals. Blood pressure was measured semiautomatically with the patients supine. Averages of an increasing number of values were calculated. Reproducibility is expressed as in Figure 2-5 (upper panel) and as a correlation between values taken one month apart. (From Mancia and colleagues [25], with permission.)

TABLE 2-1. EFFECTS ON BLOOD PRESSURE (BP) OF VERAPAMIL SLOW RELEASE (V), TRANDOLAPRIL (T), AND THE TWO DRUGS COMBINED (V+T) AFTER 8 WEEKS OF TREATMENT[*]

BP (mmHg)	Placebo (N=51)		V (N=56)		T (N=50)		V+T (N=77)	
	B	Δ	B	Δ	B	Δ	B	Δ
24-Hour SBP	142.2 ± 13.3	−0.1 ± 8.8	142.6 ± 11.0	−8.5 ± 8.9**	144.5 ± 13.7	−10.6 ± 11**	145.1 ± 15.6	−14.2 ± 10.2**†
24-Hour DBP	90.4 ± 8.4	0.2 ± 5.8	91.3 ± 7.9	−6.2 ± 5.5**	91.1 ± 8.5	−6.5 ± 7.8**	91.7 ± 9.6	−11.3 ± 6.9**†‡
Day SBP	145.6 ± 13.3	0.1 ± 9.8	146.6 ± 11.5	−9.5 ± 9.7**	148.0 ± 13.9	−11 ± 11.3**	148.8 ± 15.3	−15.2 ± 10.6**†
Day DBP	93.5 ± 8.4	0.2 ± 6.4	94.5 ± 8.2	−7 ± 6.2**	94.4 ± 8.8	−6.9 ± 8.2**	94.9 ± 9.5	−12.2 ± 7.3**†‡
Night SBP	129.8 ± 15.6	−0.3 ± 10	128.6 ± 11.4	−4.7 ± 10.8	131.9 ± 15.4	−8.9 ± 12**	131.4 ± 18.8	−10.6 ± 12.3**
Night DBP	79.4 ± 10.1	0.4 ± 8.0	79.7 ± 8.3	−3.0 ± 6.8	79.1 ± 9.5	−5 ± 8.9**	79.8 ± 12.3	−8.0 ± 9.1**†

[*]Data are shown as mean ± standard error.
**$p < .05$ vs. P.
†$p < .05$ vs. V.
‡$p < .05$ vs. T.
P = placebo; B = before; SBP = systolic blood pressure; DBP = diastolic blood pressure.

progressively increased, reaching a value similar to or greater than that of 24-hour average blood pressure (25).

COMBINATION TREATMENT

Ambulatory blood pressure monitoring is also used for testing the antihypertensive effect of combination treatment. Indeed, for combination treatment this approach is particularly indicated, because the greater reproducibility of 24-hour ambulatory blood pressure makes this value suitable to determine even small differences in the antihypertensive effect of different drug regimens. This is important because cardiovascular morbidity and mortality vary widely for a few mmHg change in systolic or diastolic blood pressure (26).

Several combinations of two drugs can be recommended for the treatment of hypertension, as emphasized by the World Health Organization/International Society of Hypertension (WHO/ISH) guidelines on antihypertensive treatment (27, 28). A combination between an ACE inhibitor and a calcium antagonist is especially appealing, however, because these two drugs have different mechanisms of action, which should make their antihypertensive efficacy additive or superior to that of the individual combination components. This was tested for the combination of trandolapril and verapamil slow release in a multicenter study with a parallel group, placebo-controlled, double-blind design that made use of ambulatory blood pressure monitoring (29). The study was conducted on mild hypertensive subjects and ambulatory blood pressure monitoring was performed (1) at the end of a washout period from previous treatment; (2) immediately after assumption of a single dose of 180 mg of verapamil slow release, 1 mg of trandolapril, or the combination of the two drugs or placebo; and (3) after 8 weeks of continuous treatment with these drugs or drug combination. As shown in Table 2-1, compared to placebo after 8 weeks of treatment either trandolapril and verapamil slow release significantly reduced 24-hour average systolic and diastolic blood pressure. The reduction was significantly greater, however, when trandolapril and verapamil were administered together, this being the case for both day (from 6:00 AM to 12:00 midnight) and night (from 12:00 midnight to 6:00 AM) blood pressure. Each treatment caused some blood pressure fall after a single-dose assumption as well, which was also greater for the combination than for the single drugs.

Thus the combination of an ACE inhibitor and a calcium antagonist has a superior antihypertensive efficacy over single combination components. Because of the possibility of greater cardiovascular protection by a blood pressure reduction below 140/90 mmHg (26), this may call for its therapeutic use in the future.

REFERENCES

1. Mancia G, Casadei R, Mutti E, et al. Ambulatory blood pressure monitoring in the evaluation of antihypertensive treatment. *Am J Med* 1989; 87(Suppl 6b):64S–69S.

2. Mancia G, Omboni S, Ravogli A, et al. Ambulatory blood pressure monitoring in the evaluation of antihypertensive treatment: additional information from a large data base. *Blood Press* 1995; 4:148–156.

3. Mancia G, Bertineri G, Grassi G, et al. Effects of blood pressure measurements by the doctor on patient's blood pressure and heart rate. *Lancet* 1983; ii:695–698.

4. Shimada K, Ogura H, Kawamoto K, et al. Noninvasive ambulatory blood pressure monitoring during clinic visit in elderly patients. *Clin Exp Hypertens* 1990; A2:151–170.

5. Parati G, Pomidossi G, Casadei R, Mancia G. Lack of alerting reactions and pressure responses to intermittent cuff inflations during noninvasive blood pressure monitoring. *Hypertension* 1985; 7:597–601.

6. Mancia G, Parati G, Pomidossi G, et al. Alerting reaction and rise in blood pressure during measurement by physician and nurse. *Hypertension* 1987; 9:209–215.

7. Parati G, Omboni S, Mancia G. Difference between office and ambulatory blood pressure and response to antihypertensive treatment. *J Hypertens* 1996; 14:(in press).

8. Mancia G, Omboni S, Parati G, et al. Lack of placebo effect on ambulatory blood pressure. *Am J Hypertens* 1995; 8:311–315.

9. Gould BA, Mann S, Davies AB, et al. Does placebo lower blood pressure? *Lancet* 1981; 2:1377–1381.

10. Dupont AG, van der Niepen P, Six RO. Placebo does not lower ambulatory blood pressure. *Br J Clin Pharmacol* 1987; 24:106–109.

11. Trazzi S, Mutti E, Frattola A, et al. Reproducibility of noninvasive and intra-arterial blood pressure monitoring: implications for studies on antihypertensive treatment. *J Hypertens* 1991; 9:115–119.

12. Conway J, Coats AJS. Ambulatory blood pressure monitoring in the design of antihypertensive drug trials. *J Hypertens* 1991; 9(Suppl 8):S57–S58.

13. Parati G, Pomidossi G, Albini F, et al. Relationship of 24-hour blood pressure mean and variability to severity of target organ damage in hypertension. *J Hypertens* 1987; 5:93–98.

14. Palatini P, Penzo M, Racioppa A, et al. Clinical relevance of night-time blood pressure and day-time blood pressure variability. *Arch Intern Med* 1992; 152:1855–1860.

15. Frattola A, Parati G, Cuspidi C, et al. Prognostic value of 24-hour blood pressure variability. *J Hypertens* 1993; 11:1133–1137.

16. Verdecchia P, Schillaci G, Guerrieri M, et al. Circadian blood pressure changes and left ventricular hypertrophy in essential hypertension. *Circulation* 1990; 81:528–536.

17. Verdecchia P, Porcellati C, Schillaci G, et al. Ambulatory blood pressure: an independent predictor of prognosis in essential hypertension. *Hypertension* 1994; 24:793–801.

18. Shimada K, Kawamoto A, Matsubayashi K, et al. Diurnal blood pressure variations and silent cerebrovascular damage in elderly patients with hypertension. *J Hypertens* 1992; 10:875–878.

19. O'Brien E, Petrie J, Littler W, et al. Short report: an outline of the revised British Hypertension Society protocol for the evaluation of blood pressure measuring devices. *J Hypertens* 1993; 11:677–679.

20. Mancia G, Parati G. Commentary on the revised British Hypertension Society protocol for evaluation of blood pressure measuring devices: a critique of aspects related to 24-hour ambulatory blood pressure measurement. *J Hypertens* 1993; 11:595–597.

21. Zanchetti A for the Italian nifedipine GITS study group, Bianchi L, Bozza M, et al. Antihypertensive effects of nifedipine GITS on clinic and ambulatory blood pressure in essential hypertensives. *High Blood Press* 1994; 3:45–56.

22. Mancia G, Omboni S, Parati G, et al. Limited reproducibility of hourly blood pressure values obtained by ambulatory blood pressure monitoring: implications for studies on antihypertensive drugs. *J Hypertens* 1992; 10:1531–1535.

23. Staessen JA, Thijs L, Mancia G, et al. Clinical trials with ambulatory blood pressure monitoring: fewer patients needed? *Lancet* 1994; 344:1552–1556.

24. Omboni S, Parati G, Zanchetti A, Mancia G. Calculation of trough:peak ratio of antihypertensive treatment from ambulatory blood pressure: methodological aspects. *J Hypertens* 1995; 10:1105–1112.

25. Mancia G, Ulian L, Parati G, Trazzi S. Increase in blood pressure reproducibility by repeated semiautomatic blood pressure measurements in the clinic environment. *J Hypertens* 1994; 12:469–473.

26. McMahon S, Peto R, Cutler J, et al. Blood pressure, stroke, and coronary heart disease. Part 1: prolonged differences in blood pressure: prospective observational studies corrected for the regression dilution bias. *Lancet* 1990; 335:765–774.

27. Guidelines sub-committee of the WHO/ISH Mild Hypertension Liaison Committee 1993. Guidelines for the management of mild hypertension: memorandum from a WHO/ISH meeting. *Hypertension* 1993; 22:392–403.

28. Mancia G, Mangoni A, Failla M, Rivolta MR. Guidelines for the treatment of hypertension: a commentary. *Curr Ther Res* 1996; 57:3–15.

29. Mancia G, Omboni S, Ravogli A, et al. Effects of verapamil (V), trandolapril (T) and their fixed combination (VT) on 24 hour blood pressure: the VeraTran study. *Am J Hypertension* 1997; (in press).

CHAPTER 3

Fixed-Dose Combinations with β-Adrenergic Blockers and Diuretics: Conventional Dose and Very-Low-Dose Formulations

William H. Frishman

The goal of drug therapy for hypertension, as with any pharmacological intervention, is to achieve the desired therapeutic response without producing toxicity—maximizing efficacy yet minimizing untoward side effects. The recommended approach advocates beginning with a low dose of a single agent, which is then titrated upward as needed (1–5). However, monotherapy is successful in only 50% to 60% of instances (6, 7) because multiple mechanisms are involved in the pathogenesis of essential hypertension, and a single drug class may not interdict all offending pathways. Also, as higher doses of individual drugs are administered, there is an increased likelihood of producing untoward side effects and stimulating the body's compensatory mechanisms that partially attenuate the incremental gain in efficacy.

Diuretics and β-adrenergic blocking drugs are the most favored first-line treatments of patients with systemic hypertension (5). They are often combined to maximize blood pressure control either as free-standing agents to be used together or in single fixed-dose combination formulations (7–11). The advantages of a single, fixed-dose combination formulation are its simplicity and convenience of use, leading to improved patient compliance and possible cost-effectiveness. The disadvantages include a reduced flexibility in dosage and a combination formulation that may be too powerful for initial therapy. However, recently there has been an interest in developing very-low-dose, fixed-dose combination formulations as initial monotherapy (12, 13) that contain low doses of a diuretic and β-blocker, such that together the drugs are effective in lowering blood pressure, but the low dose of each constituent minimizes the potential for adverse effects.

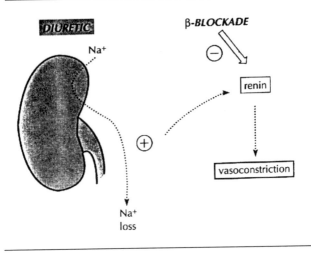

Figure 3-1. Diuretics, basically acting by sodium loss, cause an increase in circulating renin that results in angiotensin-mediated vasoconstriction. Diuretics therefore combine well with β-blockers, which inhibit the release of renin. (Adapted from Kaplan and Opie (14), with permission.)

CONVENTIONAL DOSE DIURETIC/ β-BLOCKER FORMULATIONS

Diuretics and β-blockers are excellent agents to combine in treating hypertension because together they can lower blood pressure more effectively than when either drug is used alone. The β-blocker can counteract diuretic-induced rises in plasma renin activity (14) and sympathetic nervous system outflow, while modifying diuretic-induced hypokalemia (Figure 3-1). The use of a diuretic with a β-blocker might prevent edema in patients having β-blocker-induced LV dysfunction who require better control of blood pressure.

A large number of fixed-dose diuretic/β-blocker formulations are commercially available utilizing conventional doses of thiazides (hydrochlorothiazide [HCTZ], 25 to 50 mg daily) and various β-blockers (labetalol, metoprolol, propranolol, propranolol extended release [ER], and timolol), bendroflumethiazide (5 mg with nadolol), and chlorthalidone (25 mg with atenolol) (15):

Atenolol 100 mg/chlorthalidone 25 mg
Atenolol 50 mg/chlorthalidone 25 mg

Nadolol 40 mg/bendroflumethiazide 5 mg
Nadolol 80 mg/bendroflumethiazide 5 mg

Metoprolol 100 mg/HCTZ 50 mg
Metoprolol 100 mg/HCTZ 25 mg
Metoprolol 50 mg/HCTZ 25 mg

Propranolol 40 mg/HCTZ 25 mg
Propranolol 80 mg/HCTZ 25 mg

Propranolol ER 80 mg/HCTZ 50 mg
Propranolol ER 120 mg/HCTZ 50 mg
Propranolol ER 160 mg/HCTZ 50 mg

Timolol 10 mg/HCTZ 25 mg

It is recommended that these fixed-dose formulations not be used as a first-line treatment approach in hypertension, but should be used only after each individual component is titrated to the appropriate level (it is hoped, then, a fixed-dose combination formulation will be available with the appropriate dosage determined with the monotherapy titrations).

It has been shown that diuretics and β-blockers used together are equally effective in lowering blood pressure in both black and white patients, a finding not observed when β-blockers are used as monotherapy in blacks, where they appear to be less effective than diuretic monotherapy (16).

VERY-LOW-DOSE DIURETIC/β-BLOCKER COMBINATION

Like any other product, fixed-dose combinations must be shown to be effective (i.e., superior to placebo) before Food and Drug Administration (FDA) approval (17). In addition, each component of a combination product must be shown to be contributing to the therapeutic effect desired (17). Other requirements for approval deal with adverse drug reactions. There are adverse reactions that are dose related and those that are dose independent (within the therapeutic dose range). For example, hypokalemia is an important adverse reaction with thiazide use, and this effect of diuretics is augmented as the dose is increased. It is, therefore, a dose-dependent side effect. In contrast, the cough observed with ACE inhibition can be seen with subtherapeutic doses. The FDA will grant first-line approval for a fixed-dose combination used for hypertension if the formulation contains agents that both have dose-dependent side effects or if the two agents cancel out each other's adverse reactions (18). At the same time, one has to also show that the components of a fixed-dose combination are directly additive or synergistic in their blood pressure-lowering effects (18). This can be accomplished by the use of a factorial trial (17–23) design, which involves administration of a range of two or more agents, both alone and in combination. This factorial design is also optimal for the identification of interactions because all drugs can be compared simultaneously (24–27) in the same experience. In the same experiment, from a statistical point of view, these experiments are highly efficient, for they permit precise characterization of dose-response and dose-toxicity relationships. Therefore, they also enable identification of an optimal dose ratio of the two agents in combination for purposes of both safety and effectiveness.

These criteria for first-line approval can never be granted to an ACE inhibitor combination product because cough would still be present even if the ACE inhibitor component of the combination was being used at a very low dose (18). There is a new ACE inhibitor/calcium channel blocker available that employs low doses of both components (benazepril plus amlodipine), and cough is still observed (28). A similar observation has been made with a very-low-dose combination of HCTZ 6.25 mg with benazepril.

First-line antihypertensive treatment approvals for a fixed-dose combination were recently granted to two diuretic/

TABLE 3-1. MEAN REDUCTION FROM BASELINE IN SITTING DIASTOLIC AND SYSTOLIC BLOOD PRESSURES AND RESPONSE RATES BY TREATMENT GROUP

HCTZ Dose (mg/dl)	Bisoprolol Dose (mg/dl)	# Pts.	Mean ± Standard Error Reduction in Sitting Blood Pressure at Weeks 3 to 4 (mmHg)*		% of Patients Achieving BP Goal	
			Diastolic	Systolic	Weeks 3 to 4**	Week 12†
0	0	56	3.8 ± 0.7	2.5 ± 1.2	23	24
	2.5	59	8.4 ± 0.7	9.0 ± 1.2	51	32
	10	62	10.9 ± 0.7	12.6 ± 1.2	71	47
	40	59	12.6 ± 0.7	12.6 ± 1.2	75	60
6.25	0	23	6.4 ± 0.9	6.2 ± 1.5	39	29
	2.5	28	10.8 ± 0.8	12.8 ± 1.4	61	60
	10	25	13.4 ± 0.8	16.4 ± 1.5	80	65
	40	29	15.2 ± 0.8	16.4 ± 1.4	83	77
25	0	33	8.4 ± 0.8	13.3 ± 1.4	52	44
	2.5	30	12.9 ± 0.8	19.9 ± 1.4	80	63
	10	30	15.4 ± 0.8	23.5 ± 1.4	77	78
	40	31	17.2 ± 0.8	23.5 ± 1.4	84	68

* Based on an additive model with the factors bisoprolol and hydrochlorothiazide dosage.
** Sitting diastolic blood pressure of 90 mmHg or lower, or a decrease from the baseline of 10 mmHg or more at weeks 3 to 4.
† Sitting diastolic blood pressure of 90 mmHg or lower at week 12. For the purpose of this analysis, early terminations for any reason were considered therapeutic failures.
(From Frishman and colleagues [29], with permission.)

TABLE 3-2. CONTRIBUTION OF BISOPROLOL AND HYDRO-
CHLOROTHIAZIDE TO THE REDUCTION FROM BASELINE IN
SITTING DIASTOLIC AND SYSTOLIC BLOOD PRESSURES AT
WEEKS 3 TO 4, BASED ON AN ADDITIVE MODEL

Agent	Estimated Effect on Reduction in Sitting Diastolic BP(mmHg)* Mean +/− Standard Error	p	Estimated Effect on Reduction on Sitting Systolic BP(mmHg)* Mean +/− Standard Error	p
Placebo	3.8 ± 0.7	<.01	2.5 ± 1.2	.04
Bisoprolol (mg/d)				
2.5	4.6 ± 0.9	<.01	6.6 ± 1.5	<.01
10	7.1 ± 0.9	<.01	10.2 ± 1.5	<.01
40	8.8 ± 0.9	<.01	10.2 ± 1.5	<.01
Hydrochlorothiazide (mg/d)				
6.25	2.5 ± 0.8	<.01	3.7 ± 1.3	<.01
25	4.5 ± 0.7	<.01	10.9 ± 1.3	<.01

*Based on an additive model with the factors bisoprolol dosage and hydro-
chlorothiazide dosage. Thus, for example, the estimated mean reduction in
sitting diastolic blood pressure (BP) (10.9 mmHg) for the combination of
bisoprolol 2.5 mg/d and hydrochlorothiazide 6.25 mg/d is equal to the placebo effect (3.8 mmHg) plus the effect of bisoprolol 2.5 mg/d (4.6 mmHg)
plus the effect of hydrochlorothiazide 6.25 mg/d (2.5 mmHg).
(From Frishman and colleagues [29], with permission.)

β-blocker formulations (18): low-dose chlorthalidone plus
betaxolol (not commercially available) and low-dose HCTZ
plus bisoprolol (commercially available). Both β-blockers are
β_1-selective and are combined with chlorthalidone 12.5 mg and
HCTZ 6.25 mg orally once daily.

We evaluated the low-dose HCTZ (diuretic)-bisoprolol
(β-blocker) formulation in two pivotal studies (29, 30). In the
first study, which used a factorial design (29), 512 patients
with stage I and II hypertension were randomized in a 12-
week, placebo-controlled, multicenter, 3 × 4 factorial trial
that assessed the antihypertensive effectiveness and safety
of once-daily administration of 2.5, 10, or 40 mg of bisoprolol used alone or in combination with 6.25 or 25 mg of
HCTZ. The effects of bisoprolol and HCTZ were additive
with respect to reduction in diastolic and systolic blood
pressures (Tables 3-1 and 3-2), fulfilling the first FDA requirement for first-line approval of a fixed-dose combination. The addition of HCTZ (or bisoprolol) to therapy with
bisoprolol (or HCTZ) produced an incremental reduction in
blood pressure. An HCTZ dosage of 6.25 mg daily produced
significantly less hypokalemia and less of an increase in uric
acid levels than a dosage of 25 mg daily (Table 3-3). The low-
dose combination of bisoprolol 2.5 mg daily and HCTZ 6.25
mg daily reduced diastolic blood pressure to less than 90
mmHg in 61% of patients and demonstrated a safety profile
that compared favorably with that of placebo, fulfilling the
second criteria for first-line approval: that side effects would
be reduced with the combination compared with higher
dose monotherapies that provide similar blood pressure
control to the low-dose combinations.

TABLE 3-3. MEAN CHANGE FROM BASELINE IN SERUM PO-
TASSIUM AND URIC ACID LEVELS AT WEEK 12 BY TREAT-
MENT GROUP

Hydro-chloro-thiazide (mg/d)	Bisoprolol (mg/d)	Mean change in Potassium Level (mmol/L)	Mean Change in Uric Acid Level (μmol/L)
0.0	0.0	−0.04	+10
	2.5	+0.17	+11
	10.0	+0.07	+23
	40.0	+0.12	+32
6.25	0.0	−0.05	+14
	2.5	+0.03	+8
	10.0	−0.01	+35
	40.0	−0.12	+47
25.0	0.0	−0.36	+56
	2.5	−0.28	+47
	10.0	−0.07	+45
	40.0	−0.23	+85

(From Frishman and colleagues [29], with permission.)

The second study was a confirmatory trial of 509 stage I
and II hypertensive patients using a placebo-controlled, randomized, parallel therapy design (30), that assessed the
antihypertensive effectiveness and safety of once-daily administration of 5 mg of bisoprolol used alone or in combination
with 6.25 mg of thiazide, and compared these treatments with
placebo and 25 mg HCTZ. The combination produced greater
blood pressure-lowering effects than bisoprolol 5 mg alone,
placebo, and HCTZ 25 mg, with a side effect profile of the combination comparable to placebo. Less than 1% of subjects receiving the combination developed hypokalemia (<3.4 mEq/
L) versus 6.5% on HCTZ 25 mg orally, once daily.
    Thus, the results of these studies reveal that a very-low-
dose diuretic/β-blocker formulation can be used as a first-
line monotherapy with therapeutic effects comparable to
those observed with high-dose monotherapy using either
component and with a side effect profile similar to placebo.
The low-dose combination formulation has not been evaluated in the morbidity and mortality trials that have been
done with high-dose diuretics and β-blockers in patients
with systolic and diastolic hypertension and isolated systolic hypertension. The low-dose combination appears to be
equally efficacious as an antihypertensive agent in black and
white patients, young and old patients, and men and
women (29, 30). There are no published studies describing
the additive effects of the low-dose combination formulation when added to other antihypertensive drugs (e.g., ACE
inhibitors, calcium blockers). It would be of interest to see
whether the addition of a low-dose combination formulation of ACE inhibitor to calcium blocker provides a different
blood pressure-lowering action compared with that of adding a high-dose β-blocker or high-dose diuretic.

COMPARISON OF A VERY-LOW-DOSE DIURETIC COMBINATION WITH OTHER MONOTHERAPY REGIMENS

The very-low-dose HCTZ/β-blocker combination was also compared with standard doses of other antihypertensive monotherapies in two recent studies (31).

In the first study, 218 patients with stage I and II hypertension were randomized into a placebo run-in, active-control, double-blind, dose-escalation trial comparing three once-daily doses of HCTZ/bisoprolol (6.25/2.5 mg, 6.25/5 mg, 6.25/10 mg) to amlodipine (2.5, 5, and 10 mg) and enalapril (5, 10, and 20 mg) titrated to achieve a maximal blood pressure-reducing response. Blood pressure was measured for efficacy response 24 hours after the drug dose. The study consisted of a 4- to 5-week placebo run-in phase, a 4-week dose escalation, and an 8-week maintenance phase. The study showed a comparable blood pressure-reducing effect of maximally titrated HCTZ/bisoprolol and amlodipine (–13.4/–10.7 mmHg and –12.8/–10.2 mmHg, respectively). Seventy-one percent of HCTZ/bisoprolol-treated patients and 69% of amlodipine-treated patients achieved the blood pressure goal. In contrast, enalapril caused a blood pressure reduction of –7.3/–6.6 mmHg, a significantly lower blood pressure response than that observed with amlodipine and HCTZ/bisoprolol (the enalapril effect might have been better if the drug had been used twice daily). Regarding the number of adverse experiences in the trial, there were 29 with the HCTZ/bisoprolol combination, 42 with amlodipine, and 47 with enalapril. One patient in the HCTZ/bisoprolol group dropped out because of adverse experiences versus 4 patients in each of the other groups. Finally, in this study there was mild improvement in the quality of life index that was utilized in the study with both HCTZ/bisoprolol and amlodipine, and a mild decrease with enalapril.

In the second study, 15,000 patients nationwide were randomized to receive HCTZ/bisoprolol (6.25/2.5 mg and 6.25/5 mg) or one of seven different ACE inhibitors (quinapril, ramipril, captopril, benazepril, fosinopril, enalapril, lisinopril) in an open-label practice-based study of patients with stage I and II hypertension. Drugs were titrated in dose to achieve blood pressure control over a 6-week treatment period. At the study's end, 70% of both HCTZ/bisoprolol-treated and ACE inhibitor-treated patients achieved blood pressure control (diastolic blood pressure <90 mmHg and/or a ≥10% reduction in diastolic blood pressure). Comparable efficacy was seen in both older and younger subjects, and in both men and women.

CLINICAL SITUATIONS WHERE COMBINATION DIURETIC/β-BLOCKER THERAPY CAN BE RECOMMENDED

There are no studies where dual-agent, fixed-dose combination formulations have been used to evaluate their effects on morbidity and mortality outcome in patients with systemic hypertension. The Systolic Hypertension in the Elderly Program (SHEP)(32) did include a large number of subjects who required the diuretic chlorthalidone plus atenolol to control isolated systolic hypertension, with a demonstrated morbidity benefit versus placebo. However, compared with the diuretic with comparable blood pressure control, there was no additional benefit on mortality with the combination of a diuretic and β-blocker. However, in situations where patient compliance is an issue and a diuretic and β-blocker are both needed to control blood pressure, a low-dose diuretic/β-blocker combination can be tried first, followed by a higher dose combination regimen.

SUMMARY AND CONCLUSION

Diuretics and β-blockers have been used in combination for many years and as combination, fixed-dose formulations (34). The combination has the advantage of providing greater blood pressure lowering efficacy than single drugs used alone and can negate some of the adverse reactions seen with the single drugs used alone (diuretics raise plasma renin activity and β-blockers reduce it). β-blockers have some mild antialdosterone, potassium-conserving effects that can negate the kaluretic effects of thiazides. The diuretic could also prevent edema accumulation in patients with LV dysfunction which can be aggravated by β-blockers.

Diuretics and β-blockers are also the two agents selected by the JNC-V as the best first-line treatments for hypertension based on clinical outcome data (5), so that their use in combination would be attractive. The combination would also provide greater blood pressure-lowering effects than β-blockers alone in blacks, where diuretics appear to be more effective. Combinations of diuretics and β-blockers appear to control blood pressure equally well in blacks and whites. Combinations of diuretics and β-blockers have been used in the treatment of isolated systolic hypertension in the elderly, with benefits seen on stroke, myocardial infarction, and congestive heart failure incidence when compared with placebo therapy (33).

Finally, combinations of diuretics and β-blockers have been used with very low doses of each agent to achieve blood pressure lowering effects comparable to high-dose monotherapies with a side effect profile comparable to placebo. Based on these findings, the FDA has granted a unique first-line treatment approval in hypertension for two very-low-dose combination diuretic/β-blocker formulations (HCTZ/bisoprolol and chlorthalidone/betaxolol). No other fixed-dose combination regimens for treating hypertension have received this type of approval.

REFERENCES

1. The Joint National Committee on Detection, Evaluation and Treatment of High Blood Pressure. Report of the Joint National Committee on Detection, Evaluation and Treatment of High Blood Pressure, a cooperative study. *JAMA* 1977; 237:255–261.

2. The Joint National Committee on Detection, Evaluation and Treatment of High Blood Pressure. The 1980 report of the Joint National Committee on Detection, Evaluation and Treatment of High Blood Pressure. *Arch Intern Med* 1980; 140:1280–1285.

3. The Joint National Committee on Detection, Evaluation and Treatment of High Blood Pressure. The 1984 report of the Joint National Committee on Detection, Evaluation and Treatment of High Blood Pressure. *Arch Intern Med* 1984; 144:1045–1057.

4. 1988 Joint National Committee. The 1988 report of the Joint National Committee on Detection, Evaluation and Treatment of High Blood Pressure. *Arch Intern Med* 1988; 148:1023–1038.

5. The Joint National Committee on Detection, Evaluation and Treatment of High Blood Pressure. The fifth report of the Joint National Committee on Detection, Evaluation and Treatment of High Blood Pressure (JNC-V). *Arch Intern Med* 1993: 153:154–183.

6. James IM. Which antihypertensive? *Br J Clin Pract* 1990; 44:102–105.

7. Townsend RR, Holland OB. Combination of converting enzyme inhibitor with diuretic for the treatment of hypertension. *Arch Intern Med* 1990; 150: 1175–1183.

8. Simpson FO. Combination therapy in hypertension. *Drugs* 1980; 20:69–73.

9. Enlund H, Turakka H, Tuomilehto J. Combination therapy in hypertension. *Eur J Clin Pharmacol* 1981; 21:1–8.

10. Shenfield GM. Fixed combination drug therapy. *Drugs* 1982; 23:462–480.

11. Oster JR, Epstein M. Fixed-dose combination medications for the treatment of hypertension: a critical review. *J Clin Hypertens* 1987; 3:178–193.

12. Dengler HJ, Lasagna L. Report of a workshop on fixed-ratio drug combinations. *Eur J Clin Pharmacol* 1975; 8:140–154.

13. Dollery CT. Pharmacological basis for combination therapy of hypertension. *Ann Rev Pharmacol Toxicol* 1977; 17:311–323.

14. Kaplan N, Opie LH. Antihypertensive drugs. In: Opie L, ed. *Drugs for the heart*, 4th ed. Philadelphia: W.B. Saunders, 1995: 182.

15. Frishman WH. *Current cardiovascular drugs*, 2nd ed. Philadelphia: Current Medicine, 1995: 279–280.

16. Materson BJ, Reda DJ, Cushman WL, et al. Single-drug therapy for hypertension in men. A comparison of six antihypertensive agents with placebo. *N Engl J Med* 1993; 328:914–921.

17. Division of Cardio-Renal Drug Products, FDA. Draft of the proposed guidelines for the clinical evaluation of antihypertensive drugs. Rockville, MD: FDA, 1988.

18. Fenichel RR, Lipicky RJ. Combination products as first-line pharmacotherapy. *Arch Intern Med* 1994; 154:1429–1431.

19. Goldberg MR, Rockhold FW, Offen WW. Dose-effect and concentration-effect relationships of pinacidil and hydrochlorothiazide in hypertension. *Clin Pharmacol Ther* 1989; 46:208–218.

20. Goldberg MR, Offen WW. Pinacidil with and without hydrochlorothiazide: dose-response relationships from results of a 4×3 factorial design study. *Drugs* 1988; 36(Suppl 7):83–92.

21. Burris JF, Weir MR, Oparil S, et al. An assessment of diltiazem and hydrochlorothiazide in hypertension: application of factorial trial design to a multicenter clinical trial of combination therapy. *JAMA* 1990; 263:1507–1512.

22. DeBacker G, Kornitzer M, Dramaix M, et al. The Belgian Heat Disease Prevention Project: 10-year mortality follow up. *Eur Heart J* 1988; 9:238–242.

23. Davis BR, Blaufox MD, Hawkins CM, et al. Trial of antihypertensive interventions and management. *Controlled Clin Trials* 1989; 10:11–30.

24. Snedecor GW, Cochran WG. Factorial experiments. In: *Statistical methods*. Ames, IA: Iowa State University Press, 1989: 297–332.

25. Goldberg MR, Offen WW, Rockhold FW. Factorial design: an approach to the assessment of therapeutic drug interactions in clinical trials. *J Clin Res Drug Dev* 1988; 2:215–225.

26. Pigeon JG, Copenhaver MD, Whipple JP. A method of designing clinical trials for combination drugs. *Stat Med* 1992; 2:1065–1074.

27. Chalmers TC. A potpourri of RCT topics. *Controlled Clin Trials* 1982; 3:285–298.

28. Frishman WH, Ram CVS, McMahon FG, et al. Comparison of amlodipine and benazepril monotherapy to combination therapyxin patients with systemic hypertension: a randomized, double-blind, placebo-controlled parallel group study. *J Clin Pharmacol* 1995; 35:1060–1066.

29. Frishman WH, Bryzinski BS, Coulson LR, et al. A multifactorial trial design to assess combination therapy in hypertension. *Arch Intern Med* 1994; 154:1461–1468.

30. Frishman WH, Burris JF, Mroczek WJ, et al. First-line therapy option with low-dose bisoprolol fumarate and low-dose hydrochlorothiazide in patients with stage I and stage II systemic hypertension. *J Clin Pharmacol* 1995; 35:182–188.

31. Prisant LM, Weir MR, Papademetriou V, et al. Low-dose drug combination therapy—an alternative first-line approach to hypertension treatment. *Am Heart J* 1995; 130:359–366.

32. Kostis J, Berge KG, Davis BR, et al. Effect of atenolol and reserpine on selected events in SHEP. *Am J Hypertens* 1995; 8:1147–1153.

33. SHEP Cooperative Research Group. Prevention of stroke by antihypertensive drug treatment in older persons with isolated systolic hypertension: final results of systolic hypertension in the elderly program (SHEP). *JAMA* 1991; 265:3255–3264.

34. Weber MA, Zola BE, Neutel JM. Combination drug therapy. In: Frishman WH, Sonnenblick EH (eds.). *Cardiovascular pharmacotherapeutics*. New York: McGraw Hill. 1997. In press.

CHAPTER 4

ACE Inhibitors Combined with Diuretics as Antihypertensive Therapy

Lionel H. Opie

There are important potential advantages of combining diuretics with ACE inhibitors in the therapy of hypertension (1). First, the blood pressure-lowering capacity of diuretics is limited by a reactive hyperreninemia. Therefore, the combination with ACE inhibitor therapy becomes logical and the response rate to the combination is higher, possibly over 80% in some studies.

Second, in low-renin groups such as black patients, who are often held to be a low-renin group, the response to ACE inhibition alone is poor, but the sensitivity is restored by combination with a diuretic (2).

Third, ACE inhibitors decrease the effect of angiotensin II in releasing aldosterone, so that secondary hyperaldosteronism is lessened, with a consequent tendency to potassium retention. Thiazide diuretics, on the other hand, promote potassium loss.

Fourth, the effects of thiazide diuretics in increasing blood uric acid and blood sugar are diminished by concurrent therapy with ACE inhibitors (3, 4).

Fifth, ACE inhibitors potentiate the natriuresis of diuretics. Conversely, addition of diuretics to ACE inhibitor therapy lessens the dose of ACE inhibitor required, so that the blood pressure reductions are synergistic (4).

Evidence for Improved Antihypertensive Efficacy of the Combination

There have been numerous studies showing that ACE inhibitor therapy becomes more effective in the presence of concurrent diuretic therapy (3, 5–23). Addition of a diuretic to a standard dose of ACE inhibitor gives a better response than increasing the dose of the ACE inhibitor (21). The rationale for the combination is shown in Figure 4-1.

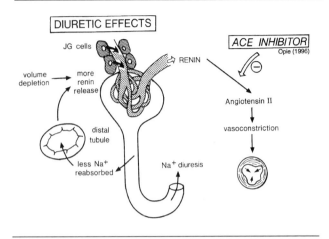

Figure 4-1. Rationale for combination of ACE inhibitors with diuretics. JG = juxtaglomerular.

Ethnic Effect

Compared with thiazide diuretics, ACE inhibitors are slightly more effective antihypertensive agents in white patients (24). In black patients, the combination ACE inhibitor plus diuretic is better than ACE inhibitor alone, with more effect on left ventricular hypertrophy (LVH) (9, 25).

Sodium Status

Sodium restriction adds to the antihypertensive efficacy of ACE inhibitor therapy (26). Even in patients already treated by captopril and a diuretic, added antihypertensive efficacy is achieved by a low-sodium diet (Figure 4-2). In simple terms, this means that patients on the ACE inhibitor plus diuretic combination therapy should, in addition, be instructed to follow a low-sodium diet.

WHAT DOSE OF THIAZIDE?

Several studies suggest that only very low doses of diuretic need be added. In a large multicenter study on 505 patients, 12.5 mg of hydrocholorothiazide decreased blood pressure as effectively when added to lisinopril 10 mg daily as did the higher dose of thiazide, namely 25 mg (28). Unfortunately, the higher dose decreased serum potassium and increased glucose levels. Thus, the addition of 12.5 mg rather than 25 mg of thiazide was clearly preferable. Likewise, a low dose (12.5 mg daily) can be as effective as a standard dose (25 mg daily) in obtaining better blood pressure control when added to enalapril 20 mg daily (29).

Yet only 6.25 mg of thiazide may be equally effective (30). In another large trial on 402 patients, hydrochlorothiazdie 6 mg or 12.5 mg was added to enalapril 20 mg daily (31). Both doses of thiazide decreased blood pressure by almost twice as much as did the ACE inhibitor alone, but the higher dose was only marginally better. Neither dose had metabolic side effects.

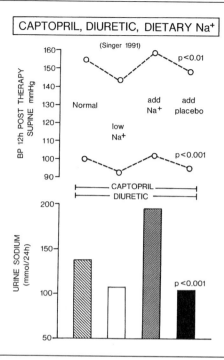

Figure **4-2.** *In patients already treated by captopril 50 mg twice daily and a diuretic, hydrochlorothiazide 25 mg once daily, a low-salt diet further reduces the blood pressure (BP) and the urine sodium. When sodium is added in the form of Slow-Sodium tablets, blood pressure increases and urine sodium rises. When Slow-Sodium placebo tablets are given, blood pressure reverts to that found with a low-sodium diet, as does urine sodium. Note the highly significant fall in urine sodium and diastolic blood pressure with sodium restriction (right-hand column, Slow-Sodium placebo). These data from Singer and colleagues (27) show that even in patients who are diuretic treated, in addition to receiving an ACE inhibitor, a low-sodium diet should be advised. (Redrawn from the data of Singer and colleagues [27] with permission.)*

Unfortunately, two other large trials with a more sensitive factorial design, one with quinapril (32) and another with ramipril (4), show that a thiazide dose of not less than 25 mg was required to achieve optimal blood pressure lowering. In both cases the lowest dose of the ACE inhibitor attenuated the hypokalemia induced by the diuretic. Thus the question of the optimal diuretic for the combination is still up in the air.

Nonetheless, taking together the results of the 1,007 patients from the standard randomized studies and the 994 patients from the factorial studies, the optimal way to start may be with low doses of the ACE inhibitor (e.g., ramipril 2.5 mg, enalapril 5 mg, or lisinopril 10 mg) and of the diuretic (6 to 12.5 mg), and then doubling both.

METABOLIC EFFECTS OF THIAZIDE AND ACE INHIBITOR: INSULIN RESISTANCE

Insulin resistance is associated with increased cardiovascular risk in hypertensive patients (33) and in those with LVH (34). Whereas ACE inhibitors tend to decrease insulin resistance (35), diuretics tend to increase insulin resistance as shown in an influential study by Pollare and colleagues (36). These authors achieved equal blood pressure reduction in a group of patients with initial values of about 165/100 mmHg, using approximately a mean dose of captopril 80 mg daily and of hydrochlorothiazide 40 mg daily. Over the 4-month treatment period, captopril appeared to increase the sensitivity to infused insulin, whereas hydrochlorothiazide appeared to decrease it. Hydrochlorothiazide also increased serum cholesterol and triglyceride levels. No outcome data were presented to indicate that these adverse metabolic effects had hard end points such as a greater incidence of diabetes mellitus or coronary heart disease. Nonetheless, on first principles, the changes found during thiazide therapy could with justification be regarded as disadvantageous (33).

A major reservation attached to the Pollare study (36) is that the dose of hydrochlorothiazide (mean daily dose about 40 mg) is considerably higher than that currently recommended for thiazide monotherapy, which should begin at 6.25 mg and be no more than 25 mg daily (37). Such low diuretic doses may not, in practice, be adequately antihypertensive (32). Thus, there is a logical argument for the use of low-dose diuretic combined with ACE inhibitors to lessen the trend to insulin resistance, as shown by the increased blood glucose levels when 25 mg of thiazide but not 12.5 mg daily was added to lisinopril (28). Nonetheless, there appear to be no formal studies relating added diuretic dose to measured insulin resistance.

Potential Disadvantages of the Combination ACE Inhibitor-Diuretics

There are several potential problems with this type of combination therapy. First, when there is marked salt retention, as in severe heart failure but seldom in hypertension, there tends to be a considerable reactive hyperreninemia, so that the ACE inhibitor can cause a serious hypotensive first-dose effect. An analogous situation in hypertension could be the severe fall in blood pressure that may be induced by an ACE inhibitor when given to a patient with renal artery stenosis. This problem can be anticipated by giving a very low first dose of the ACE inhibitor as a test dose, for example 6.25 mg of captopril, to all patients being evaluated for ACE inhibitor therapy.

Second, the addition of an ACE inhibitor to a diuretic may decrease renal function in patients with resistant heart failure (38) or in those with severe hypertension and a fixed renal vascular resistance, as in the case of bilateral renal artery stenosis. The latter situation is therefore a contraindication to ACE inhibitor therapy for hypertension. In the case of severe heart failure, patients need monitoring for some days after the addition of ACE inhibitor therapy and careful dose titration.

Third, when combined with potassium-sparing diuretics or potassium supplements, there is danger of hyperkalemia, especially in the added presence of renal impairment

(39). The ideal diuretic to be combined with an ACE inhibitor should not have any potassium-retaining qualities nor have any built-in or added potassium supplementation (40). A standard combination could be the usual dose of the ACE inhibitor together with a low-dose diuretic (12.5 mg or less hydrochlorothiazide daily).

Fourth, there appears to be a specific inhibitory effect of captopril on the diuretic action of furosemide, because captopril interferes with the renal tubular excretion of furosemide (41). The result is a marked loss of the natriuretic and diuretic effects of furosemide (42). This negative interaction is not shared by enalapril (43) nor by ramipril (41) nor by ultra-low-dose captopril (44). Therefore, at least in the case of captopril when used for hypertension, combination with diuretic therapy should not be by furosemide but by a thiazide.

IS A DIURETIC REQUIRED MORE OFTEN WITH AN ACE INHIBITOR THAN WITH A BETA-BLOCKER?

In the landmark "quality of life" study of Croog and colleagues (12), captopril 50 mg twice daily was the approximate antihypertensive equivalent of propranolol 80 mg twice daily (160 mg daily) on diastolic blood pressure. Systolic values were not reported. It is well known that the study found that captopril caused fewer side effects than did propranolol and in fact improved the quality of life, whereas propranolol did not. It is less well known that added diuretic therapy by hydrochlorothiazide 25 to 50 mg daily was required to control the blood pressure in 33% of captopril-treated patients and only 22% of propranolol-treated patients (p < 0.02). The inescapable conclusion must be that for monotherapy in hypertension, captopril is less effective than propranolol, but propranolol induces more side effects. Thus, patients felt better on captopril alone than on propranolol, but their blood pressure values were higher. The addition of the diuretic to captopril, to achieve equal blood pressure reduction, altered the quality of life: "improvement in the score on the general well-being index was substantially reduced " (12, p.1661). Logically, the quality of life would be less impaired with the addition of low- rather than high-dose diuretic therapy.

ACE INHIBITION PLUS DIURETIC AS PART OF TRIPLE THERAPY

Blood pressures may not respond to dual combination therapy. When, for example, blood pressure reduction has already been attempted with the combination of a calcium antagonist (amlodipine) and an ACE inhibitor (lisinopril), then the further addition of a diuretic is more effective than adding a beta-blocker (45). This finding may not be surprising in view of the studies showing that there is no good hypotensive effect of adding a beta-blocker to an ACE inhibitor (see references in Antonios and colleagues [45]).

CONCLUSIONS

Because ACE inhibitor therapy and diuretics as monotherapy are relatively ineffective in certain population groups, and because sodium restriction is required for better expression of the effects of ACE inhibition on the blood pressure, a combination of therapy by these two types of agents is very logical. The combination is also metabolically safe provided that a low dose of thiazide is used. Just what the ideal low dose would be for any given patient depends on a number of factors, including ethnic group and age, and cannot be predicted with accuracy from existing data. Thus, if a fixed dose of ACE inhibitor and a diuretic should be used, but without total success, then there should first be combination with a low-salt diet, and then the diuretic dose could be increased. Before determining that any of these combinations do not work, it should be recalled that diuretic therapy may take 6 to 12 weeks to become fully effective (45).

REFERENCES

1. Johnston DL, Lesoway R, Humen DP, Kostuk WJ. Clinical and hemodynamic evaluation of propranolol in combination with verapamil, nifedipine and diltiazem in exertional angina pectoris: a placebo-controlled, double-blind, randomized, cross-over study. *Am J Cardiol* 1985; 55:680–687.

2. Veterans Administration Cooperative Study Group on Antihypertensive Agents. Captopril: evaluation of low doses, twice-daily doses and the addition of diuretic for the treatment of mild to moderate hypertension. *Clin Sci* 1982; 14:127–131.

3. Weinberger MH. Comparison of captopril and hydrochlorothiazide alone and in combination in mild to moderate essential hypertension. *Br J Clin Pharmacol* 1982; 14:127–131.

4. Scholze J, Group for the East Germany Collaborative Trial. Short report: ramipril and hydrochlorothiazide combination therapy in hypertension: a clinical trial of factorial design. *J Hypertens* 1993; 11:217–221.

5. MacGregor GA, Markandu ND, Banks RA, et al. Captopril in essential hypertension; contrasting effects of adding hydrochlorothiazide or propranolol. *Br Med J* 1982; 284:693–696.

6. Weinberger MH. Influence of an angiotensin-converting enzyme inhibitor on diuretic-induced metabolic effects in hypertension. *Hypertension* 1983; 5:132–138.

7. Vlasses PH, Rotmensch HH, Swanson BN, et al. Comparative antihypertensive effects of enalapril maleate and hydrochlorothiazide, alone and in combination. *J Clin Pharmacol* 1983; 23:227–233.

8. Thind GS, Mahaptra RK, Johnson A, Coleman RD. Low-dose captopril tritration in patients with moderate-to-severe hypertension treated with diuretics. *Circulation* 1983; 67:1340–1346.

9. Vidt DG. A controlled multiclinic study to compare the antihypertensive effects of MK-421, hydrochlorothiazide, and MK-421 combined with hydrochlorothiazide in patients with mild to moderate essential hypertension. *J Hypertens* 1984; 2:227–233.

10. Bauer JH, Jones LB. Comparative studies: enalapril versus hydrochlorothiazide as first-step therapy for the treatment of primary hypertension. *Am J Kidney Dis* 1984; 4:55–62.

11. Freier PA, Wollam GL, Hall WD, et al. Blood pressure plasma volume and catecholamine levels during analapril therapy in blacks with hypertension. *Clin Pharmacol Ther* 1984; 36:731–737.

12. Croog SH, Levine S, Testa MA, et al. The effect of antihypertensive therapy on the quality of life. *N Engl J Med* 1986; 314:1657–1664.

13. Merrill DD, Byymy RL, Carr A, et al. Lisonopril/TCTZ in essential hypertension [abstract]. *Clin Pharmacol Ther* 1987; 41:227.

14. Muiesan G, Agabiti-Rosei E, Buoninconti R. Antihypertensive efficacy and tolerability of captopril in elderly: comparison with hydrochlorothiazide and placebo in a multicentre double-blind study. *J Hypertens* 1987; 2:89–92.

15. Shapiro DL, Liss CL, Walker JF, et al. Enalapril and hydrochlorothiazide as antihypertensive agents in the elderly. *J Cardiovasc Pharmacol* 1987; 10:S160–S162.

16. Frishman WH, Goldberger J, Sherman D. Enalapril, hydrochlorothiazide and combination therapy in patients with moderate hypertension. *J Clin Hypertens* 1987; 3:520–527.

17. Kayanakis JG, Baulac L. The comparative study of once-daily administration of captopril 50 mg, hydrochlorothiazide 25 mg and their combination in mild to moderate hypertension. *Br J Clin Pharmacol* 1987; 23:89S–92S.

18. Kochar MS, Bolek G, Klabfleisch JH, Olzinski P. A 52 week comparison of lisinopril, hydrochlorothiazide and their combination in hypertension. *J Clin Pharmacol* 1987; 27:373–377.

19. Zezulka AV, Gill JS, Dews I. Comparison of enalapril and bendrofluazide for treatment of systemic hypertension. *Am J Cardiol* 1987; 59:630–633.

20. Gums JG, Lopez MN, Quay GP, et al. Comparative evaluation of enalapril and hydrochlorothiazide in elderly patients with mild to moderate hypertension. *Drug Intell Clin Pharmacol* 1988; 22:680–684.

21. Sassano P, Chatellier G, Billaud E, et al. Comparison of increase in the enalapril dose and addition of hydrochlorothizide as second-step treatment of hypertensive patients not controlled by enalapril alone. *J Cardiovasc Pharmacol* 1989; 13:314–319.

22. Zanchetti A, Desche P. Perindopril. First-line treatment for hypertension. *Clin Exp Ther Pract* 1989; A11;555–573.

23. Brown CL, Backhouse CI, Grippat JC, Santoni JP. The effect of perindopril and hydrochlorothiazide alone and in combination on blood pressure and on the renin-angiotensin system in hypertensive subjects. *Eur J Clin Pharmacol* 1990; 39:327–332.

24. Perry IJ, Beevers DG. ACE inhibitors compared with thiazide diuretics as first-step antihypertensive therapy. *Cardiovasc Drugs Ther* 1989; 3:815–819.

25. Pool JL, Gennari J, Goldstein R, et al. Controlled multicentre study of antihypertensive effects of lisinopril, hydrochlorothiazide and lisinopril plus hydrochlorothiazide in the treatment of 394 patients with mild to moderate essential hypertension. *J Cardiovasc Pharmacol* 1987; 9:S36–S42.

26. Morgan T, Anderson A. Clinical efficacy of perindopril in hypertension. *Pharmacol Physiol* 1992; 19:61–65.

27. Singer DRJ, Markandu ND, Sugden AI, et al. Sodium restriction in hypertensive patients treated with a converting enzyme inhibitor and a thiazide. *Hypertension* 1991; 17:798–803.

28. Chrysant SG, The Lisinopril-Hydrochlorothiazide Group. Antihypertensive effectiveness of low-dose hydrochlorothiazide combination. A large multicenter study. *Arch Intern Med* 1994; 154:737–743.

29. Dahlöf B, Andren L, Eggertsen R, et al. Potentiation of the anti-hypertensive effect of enalapril by randomised addition of different doses of hydrochlorothiazide. *J Hypertens* 1985; 3:S483–S486.

30. Andren L, Weiner L, Svensson A, Hanson L. Enalapril with either a "very low" or "low" dose of hydrochlorothiazide is equally effective in essential hypertension. A double-blind trial in 100 hypertensive patients. *J Hypertens* 1983; 1:384–386.

31. Guul SJ, Os I, Jounela AJ. The efficacy and tolerability of enalapril in a formulation with a very low dose of hydrochlorothiazide in hypertensive patients resistant to enalapril monotherapy. *Am J Hypertens* 1995; 8:727–731.

32. Canter D, Frank GH, Knapp LK, et al. Quinapril and hydrochlorothiazide combination for control of hypertension: assessment by factorial design. *J Hum Hypertens* 1994; 8:155–162.

33. Reaven GM, Lithell H, Landsberg L. Hypertension and associated metabolic abnormalities—the role of insulin resistance and the sympathoadrenal system. *N Engl J Med* 1996; 334:374–381.

34. Lind L, Andersson P, Andren L, et al. Left ventricular hypertrophy in hypertension is associated with the insulin resistance metabolic syndrome. *J Hypertens* 1995; 13:433–438.

35. Paolisso G, Bambardella A, Verza M, et al. ACE inhibition improves insulin-sensitivity in aged insulin-resistant hypertensive patients. *J Hum Hypertens* 1992; 6:175–179.

36. Pollare T, Lithell H, Berne C. A comparison of the effects of hydrochlorothiazide and captopril on glucose and lipid metabolism in patients with hypertension. *N Engl J Med* 1989; 321:868–873.

37. Kaplan NM, Opie LH. Antihypertensive drugs. In: Opie L, ed. *Drugs for the heart*. Philadelphia: W.B. Saunders, 1995: 174–205.

38. Dargie J, Cleland J, Findlay I, et al. Combination of verapamil and β-blockers in systemic hypertension. *Am J Cardiol* 1986; 57:80D–82D.

39. Textor SC, Bravo EL, Fouad FM, Tarazi RC. Hyperkalaemia in azotemic patients during angiotensin-converting enzyme inhibition and aldosterone reduction with captopril. *Am J Med* 1982; 73:719–725.

40. Burnakis TG, Mioduch HJ. Combined therapy with captopril and potassium supplementation. A potential for hyperkalemia. *Arch Intern Med* 1984; 144:2371–2372.

41. Toussaint C, Masselink A, Gentges A, et al. Interference of different ACE inhibitors with the diuretic action of furosemide and hydrochlorothiazide. *Klin Wochenschr* 1989; 67:1138–1146.

42. McLay JS, McMurray JJ, Bridges AB. Acute effects of furosemide in patients with chronic heart failure. *Am Heart J* 1993; 126:879–886.

43. van Hecken AM, Verbesselt R, Buntinx A, et al. Absence of a pharmacokinetic interaction between enalapril and furosemide. *Br J Clin Pharmacol* 1987; 23:84–87.

44. Motwani JG, Fenwick MK, Morton JJ, Struthers AD. Furosemide-induced natriuresis is augmented by ultra-low dose captopril but not by standard doses of captopril in chronic heart failure. *Circulation* 1992; 86:439–445.

45. Antonios TF, Cappuccio FP, Markandu ND, et al. A diuretic is more effective than a β-blocker in hypertensive patients not controlled on amlodipine and lisinopril. *Hypertension* 1996; 27:1325–1328.

CHAPTER 5

Diuretics and Angiotensin Receptor Inhibitors

Ehud Grossman
Franz H. Messerli
Michael A. Weber

The renin-angiotensin system (RAS) participates in the regulation of blood pressure and fluid and electrolyte balance. Activation of this system results in formation of angiotensin II (AII). The effects of AII at the type I receptor (AT_1) produce physiological consequences critical to cardiovascular homeostasis, including vasoconstriction, sodium/fluid retention, augmentation of the sympathetic activity, cellular growth, and positive inotropic effects. The RAS has been shown to participate in the pathogenesis of systemic hypertension and congestive heart failure (CHF)(1, 2). Therefore, blocking this system may lower blood pressure and improve heart failure. Inhibition of AII activity at the receptor site is one of the ways to block the renin-angiotensin system. The first known antagonists of AII at its receptor were peptide analogs of AII. However, the short action, poor bioavailability, and partial agonistic properties limited the use of these peptides as therapeutic agents. The breakthrough came with the discovery of the nonpeptide AII receptor antagonists that have good oral bioavailability and lack agonistic properties. The prototype of this group is losartan potassium (DuP 753) that has been recently approved for use in the treatment of hypertension in Scandinavia, the United Kingdom, several European countries, and the United States. This chapter will review the efficacy and tolerability of AII receptor antagonists in combination with diuretics. Since the literature related to AII receptor antagonists so far deals mainly with losartan potassium, we will focus this discussion on losartan potassium, but we assume that the information is relevant for the other AII receptor antagonists that will be available in the future.

PHARMACOKINETIC PROPERTIES

The AT_1 receptor antagonists being developed are phenyl tetrazole-substituted imidazoles. Several AT_1 receptor antagonists are in clinical development (Table 5-1). Some are

TABLE 5-1. ANGIOTENSIN II ANTAGONISTS UNDERGOING
CLINICAL INVESTIGATION PUBLISHED CLINICAL REPORTS*

Compound	Regulatory Phase	Oral Dose mg†	Manufacturer/Sponsor
Losartan (DuP 753)	IV	50	DuPont Merck
Eprosartan (SK&F 108566)	II-III	150–350	SmithKline Beecham
Candesartan (TCV 116)	III	5–10	Takeda and Astra
Irbesartan (SR 47436)	III	10–50	Sanofi and Bristol-Myers Squibb
Zolarsartan (GR 117289C)	II‡	?	Glaxo
Telmisartan (BIBR 0277 SE)	II-III	40–80	Boeringer Ingelheim
Tasosartan (ANA 756)	III	>100	Wyeth-Ayerst
Valsartan (CGP 48933)	III	>100	Novartis

*Adapted from Wexler et al. (55).
†Based on antagonism of angiotensin II pressor effects and/or (if available) antihypertensive activity. Question mark indicates data unknown.
‡Development suspended.

active as they are and some are prodrugs that are converted to active metabolites. Pharmacologically, AT_1 receptor antagonists block the pressor and other functional responses to AII both in vitro and in vivo. Unlike the peptide antagonist saralasin, the nonpeptide AT_1 receptor antagonists display no intrinsic agonistic properties.

The prototype AT_1 receptor antagonist losartan potassium is oxidized in the liver to yield the pharmacologically active carboxylic acid metabolite E3174 (3, 4). Oral bioavailability of losartan potassium is approximately 33% and is unaffected by food (5). Peak plasma concentrations (C_{max}) of a single dose of losartan potassium are dose proportional within the range of 25 to 200 mg. Time to achieve C_{max} is reported as 0.7 to 1.3 hours for losartan potassium and 2 to 3 hours for E3174. Multiple-dose (7-day) administration does not appear to alter significantly the pharmacokinetics of losartan potassium or E3174.

Losartan potassium was undetectable in plasma at 10 hours postdose, whereas E3174 was measurable at 24 hours (6). Plasma concentrations of E3174 in healthy volunteers correlated more closely with pressor response than did those of the parent compound (7). Antihypertensive effects were dose dependent within the range 40 to 120 mg and reached a plateau at E3174 concentrations of about 200 µg/L (7).

Both compounds are highly protein bound (>98%); the volume of distribution is 34 L for losartan potassium and 12 L for the metabolite (5). In rats, losartan potassium crossed the blood-brain barrier after a single intravenous dose (8) but, of more clinical importance, not after single or multiple oral doses (9). The drug did not cross the placenta in a sheep experiment (10), but this model may not be applicable to humans. Like ACE inhibitors, losartan potassium is contraindicated in pregnancy.

METABOLISM AND ELIMINATION

In most individuals about 14% of a dose of losartan potassium is converted by cytochrome P4503A to the active metabolite E3174 (5, 11). The terminal elimination half-life is longer for E3174 (about 4 to 10 hours) than for losartan potassium (about 2 hours). Renal clearance is 5.6 L/hr for losartan potassium 50 mg and about 1.5 L/hr for its metabolite (6). About 35% of a radiolabeled oral dose is recovered in the urine and 65% in the feces (5). Less than 5% of a losartan potassium dose is excreted unchanged in the urine in patients with normal renal function (12). Renal impairment only slightly changed plasma concentrations of losartan potassium and E3174, but the changes were not considered to be clinically important (12). On the other hand, in patients with cirrhosis, plasma concentrations of losartan potassium and E3174 increased 5-fold and 1.7-fold, respectively; oral bioavailability was doubled; and total plasma clearance was halved (5). Dosage adjustment is therefore required in this population.

PHARMACODYNAMIC PROPERTIES

Losartan potassium is highly and specifically bound to AT_1 receptors. The active metabolie E3174 has 10-fold greater affinity for AT_1 receptors and is estimated to be approximately 15 to 20 times more potent than its parent compound (11).

Binding of losartan potassium to the AT_1 receptor is saturable, reversible, and competitive (13), whereas the metabolite is a noncompetitive antagonist, causing nonparallel shifts to the right of the concentration-contractile response curve. The drug competitively blocked AII-induced contraction of rabbit aorta, guinea pig ileum, and rat uterus (14, 15). In healthy volunteers oral administration of losartan potassium blocked the vasoconstrictor and pressor responses to exogenous angiotensin I (AI) and AII (16, 17). The drug and its active metabolite E3174 had no AII agonist effects in the concentrations tested.

Blockade of AT_1 receptors is the basis for losartan potassium application in patients with hypertension. Clinical evidence (18–20) indicates that losartan potassium is also likely to be beneficial in patients with CHF.

HEMODYNAMIC EFFECTS

Losartan reduces systolic and diastolic blood pressure through a decrease in peripheral resistance without a change in heart rate and cardiac output. The hypotensive effect lasts 24 hours and therefore losartan potassium can be used as a once-daily drug. Its long duration activity was confirmed by 24-hour ambulatory blood pressure monitoring (21) and by placebo-adjusted trough-to-peak ratios of greater than 50% for the 50- to 100-mg dose.

EFFECTS ON RENAL HEMODYNAMICS AND FUNCTION

Losartan potassium maintained renal blood flow, glomerular filtration rate (GFR), and urine volume unchanged. Excretion of urinary sodium and potassium in healthy individuals on a low-salt diet was either increased (22) or unchanged (23). Hyperkalemia has been reported infrequently in clinical trials.

Inconsistent results have been described regarding the effect of losartan potassium on uric acid excretion (22, 24–27). While some studies demonstrated a significant uricosuria with losartan potassium (22, 25, 27), others failed to do so (24, 26). Irbesartan, another angiotensin II antagonist, exerted no uricosuric effect in hypertensive patients (28), suggesting that the uricosuric effect may be unrelated to AT_1 receptor blockade. It has been shown that losartan potassium lowered proteinuria in otherwise healthy hypertensive patients, in patients with renal failure (29, 30), and in elderly patients with or without noninsulin-dependent diabetes mellitus (NIDDM)(31).

METABOLIC AND NEUROENDOCRINE EFFECTS

Losartan potassium does not adversely affect lipid profile and insulin sensitivity in nondiabetic patients with hypertension (24,32). In some small studies losartan even improved lipid profile and insulin sensitivity (33–35). The effects of losartan potassium on the renin-angiotensin system are consistent with inhibition of AII. In healthy volunteers, losartan potassium increased plasma renin activity and plasma AII levels, but produced inconsistent effects on plasma aldosterone levels (17, 22, 23, 36). In patients with essential hypertension, plasma aldosterone levels fell by 58% after 6 weeks of therapy with the 100-mg/day dosage (37) and by 17% after a month's treatment with losartan potassium 50 mg/day (24). Plasma renin activity and plasma AII levels increased after losartan and irbesartan therapy (24, 28, 37). The peak increase was observed at about 2 weeks after therapy and declined thereafter (24). Losartan potassium does not stimulate the sympathetic nervous system, as the plasma levels of adrenaline and noradrenaline do not increase or even decrease during treatment (24, 37). Another AT_1 receptor antagonist, TCV-116, also does not stimulate the sympathetic nervous system as judged by changes in response to a stress test and a cold pressor test or by muscle sympathetic nerve activity (38).

CLINICAL EFFICACY OF AT_1 RECEPTOR ANTAGONISTS IN HYPERTENSION

Losartan potassium in the 50-mg/day dosage has proved to be efficacious and superior to placebo in large placebo-controlled trials (11). Increasing the dose to 100 mg daily does not seem to elicit any additional benefit (39, 40). The antihypertensive effect of losartan potassium is evident within 2 weeks of starting treatment and is maximized at 3 to 6 weeks after treatment initiation. The activity of the renin-angiotensin system determines the response to losartan, as Tsunoda and colleagues (25) found that losartan was less effective in patients with low-renin hypertension, and Grossman and associates (24) found that the decrease in blood pressure was related to the baseline and the change in plasma renin activity.

In a few comparative studies, losartan potassium was equipotent to ACE inhibitors, hydrochlorothiazide, atenolol, and extended-release felodipine (41–45). Losartan potassium is effective in elderly hypertensive patients. In one study (42) conducted in elderly patients, losartan potassium was as effective as extended-release felodipine. Dahlof and coworkers (41) also found no differences in response to losartan potassium between younger and elderly patients. It is not yet known whether responses to losartan are affected by factors such as ethnicity and gender. Losartan potassium is well tolerated and only few side effects are drug related. In a recent study (46) of data obtained from more than 2,900 hypertensive patients, losartan potassium monotherapy produced an incidence of drug-related adverse events (15.3% versus 15.5%) and patient withdrawal (2.3% versus 3.7%) that was similar to placebo. Drug-related events experienced most frequently with losartan potassium were headache (4.2%), asthenia/fatigue (2%), and dizziness, which was the only drug-related event reported more frequently with losartan potassium than with placebo (2.4% versus 1.3%). When a causal relationship of events to treatment was not considered, the most commonly reported unwanted events in patients receiving losartan potassium monotherapy were headache (14.1%), upper respiratory tract infection (6.5%), dizziness (4.1%), asthenia/fatigue (3.8%), and cough (3.1%). The incidence of edema with losartan was 1.7%, a rate similar to that for placebo (1.9%). Orthostatic effects and first-dose hypotension appear uncommon, occurring in less than 0.5% of losartan potassium 25- to 50-mg recipients and 2.2% of 100-mg recipients. There is a case report of a patient who developed angioedema during losartan potassium therapy (47). Dose, age, gender, and race are reported to have no influence on the tolerability profile of losartan potassium; quantitative data for between-group comparisons are unavailable. Unlike the ACE inhibitors, losartan potassium does not provoke cough. In a study that was designed specifically to assess the incidence and severity of cough in patients with a history of cough during ACE inhibitor therapy, losartan was less than half as likely as the ACE inhibitor lisinopril to provoke cough (45). The incidence of spontaneously reported cough was 3.1% during treatment with losartan potassium, compared to 8.8% with ACE inhibitors and 2.6% with placebo (46).

There are only a few published studies on other AII receptor antagonists in hypertension. In an open clinical trial (48), TCV-116 showed dose-dependent cumulative efficacy of 15% for 1 mg/day, 38% for 2 mg/day, 60% for 4 mg/day, and 76% for 8 mg/day. Another study (28) was of a double-blind parallel group in which irbesartan 100 mg gave a satisfactory fall in blood pressure over 24 hours without change in heart rate. A preliminary report (49) on 17 patients suggests that TCV-116 is relatively safe in the elderly.

COMBINATION OF ANGIOTENSIN RECEPTOR INHIBITOR AND DIURETICS

Less than 50% of hypertensive patients will achieve goal blood pressure (<140/90 mmHg) with losartan potassium 50 mg daily as monotherapy (24, 43, 50). Most of these patients will require the addition of other antihypertensive agents (51). A combination of hydrochlorothiazide and AT_1 receptor antagonist should produce an additive hypotensive effect, because the two classes of drugs have complementary and different pharmacological mechanisms of action. Thiazide diuretics increase plasma renin activity and AT_1 receptor antagonists are more effective in hypertensive patients with high renin. Indeed, few studies evaluated the efficacy, safety, and tolerability of a combination of low-dose hydrochlorothiazide and losartan potassium in hypertensive patients. Soffer and colleagues (52) added losartan potassium to hydrochlorothiazide in hypertensive patients whose blood pressure was not adequately controlled by 25 mg hydrochlorothiazide monotherapy. After a 4-week monotherapy period of 25 mg hydrochlorothiazide, 304 patients with trough, sitting diastolic blood pressure between 93 and 120 mmHg were maintained on 25 mg hydrochlorothiazide and randomized double-blind into treatment arms consisting of either 25, 50, or 100 mg losartan or placebo once daily for 12 weeks. The addition of all doses of losartan potassium to hydrochlorothiazide produced a significant decrease in blood pressure 1 week after randomization. The antihypertensive response was greater at week 3 than at week 1, with some additional decrease in blood pressure in some groups in later time. Weber and associates (40) added hydrochlorothiazide 12.5 mg daily for 2 weeks to patients whose clinical diastolic blood pressure remained at 85 mmHg or higher during losartan potassium monotherapy. They found that the addition of hydrochlorothiazide lowered diastolic blood pressure by a further 6.1 to 7.8 mmHg, similar to the decrease of 6.4 mmHg in the placebo plus hydrochlorothiazide group. Adding hydrochlorothiazide in doses greater than 12.5 mg to losartan potassium 50 mg reduced diastolic blood pressure by an additional 4 to 6 mmHg versus monotherapy with losartan potassium 50 mg (51, 53). Grossman and colleagues studied the long-term effects of losartan potassium in a small group of hypertensive patients (24). After 4 weeks of treatment with losartan potassium 50 mg daily, hydrochlorothiazide was added for 12 months to those patients whose sitting diastolic blood pressure remained 93 mmHg or higher. The addition of hydrochlorothiazide further decreased blood pressure.

In patients with severe hypertension, a combination of losartan potassium and hydrochlorothiazide has provided a satisfactory response in about one-third of the patients (43, 54). MacKay and colleagues (50) compared in a double-blind study of 12 weeks the effects of losartan 50 mg daily, hydrochlorothiazide, concomitant therapy with losartan and one of two doses of hydrochlorothiazide, and placebo. The combination of losartan potassium 50 mg daily and very-low-dose hydrochlorothiazide (6.25 mg daily) was not superior to losartan potassium alone. However, the combination of 50 mg of losartan potassium and 12.5 mg of hydrochlorothiazide produced a reduction in blood pressure that was significantly greater than that of the individual components. Seventy-eight percent of the patients treated with 50 mg of losartan and 12.5 mg of hydrochlorothiazide had an excellent or good antihypertensive response. The peak-to-trough placebo-adjusted ratio for the combination of losartan 50 mg and hydrochlorothiazide 12.5 mg was 85%, indicating a smooth reduction in blood pressure that was sustained over 24 hours.

Metabolic Effects and Safety

Since losartan potassium produces a uricosuric effect, the addition of losartan potassium to hydrochlorothiazide blunts the increase in serum uric acid levels seen with hydrochlorothiazide alone. Like ACE inhibitors, losartan attenuates the decrease in serum potassium observed with hydrochlorothiazide alone. The combination of losartan potassium 50 mg daily and hydrochlorothiazide 12.5 mg daily displays an excellent safety profile. In a recent study (50) there were no statistically significant differences in adverse experiences in patients receiving 50 mg of losartan potassium and 12.5 mg of hydrochlorothiazide compared with those receiving placebo.

CONCLUSIONS

The nonpeptide AII receptor antagonists belong to a new class of drugs that lower blood pressure by blocking the renin-angiotensin-aldosterone system at the receptor site. These agents are equipotent to ACE inhibitors in lowering blood pressure with fewer side effects. The prototype of this class is losartan potassium (DuP 753), which has been recently approved for use in the treatment of hypertension in Scandinavia, the United Kingdom, several European countries, and the United States. The recommended dose of losartan potassium is 50 mg once daily. If losartan alone is not sufficient to control blood pressure, the addition of hydrochlorothiazide 12.5 mg once daily is recommended. The combination of hydrochlorothiazide and angiotensin II receptor antagonist produces an additive hypotensive effect, because the two classes of drugs have complementary and different pharmacological mechanisms of action. This combination displays an excellent safety profile with a low rate of adverse events. Moreover, this combination blunts the increase in serum uric acid and the decrease in serum potassium levels seen with hydrochlorothiazide alone.

REFERENCES

1. Laragh JH, Baer L, Brunner HR, et al. Renin, angiotensin and aldosterone system in pathogenesis and management of hypertensive vascular disease. *Am J Med* 1972; 52:633–652.

2. Curtis C, Cohn JN, Vrobel T, Franciosa JA. Role of the renin-angiotensin system in the systemic vasoconstriction of chronic congestive heart failure. *Circulation* 1978; 58:763–770.

3. Stearns RA, Miller RR, Doss GA, et al. The metabolism of DuP753, a nonpeptide angiotensin II receptor antagonist, by rat, monkey, and human liver slices. *Drug Metab Dispos* 1992; 20:281–287.

4. Wong PC, Price WA, Chiu AT, et al. Nonpeptide angiotensin II receptor antagonists. XI. Pharmacology of EXP3174: an active metabolite of DuP735, an orally active antihypertensive agent. *J Pharmacol Exp Ther* 1990; 255:211–217.

5. Merck & Co., Inc. *Losartan potassium prescribing information.* West Point, PA: Merck & Co., 1995.

6. Ohtawa M, Takayama F, Saitoh K. Pharmacokinetics and biochemical efficacy after single and multiple oral administration of losartan, an orally active nonpeptide angiotensin II receptor antagonist, in humans. *Br J Clin Pharmacol* 1993; 35:290-297,

7. Munafo A, Christen Y, Nussberger J, et al. Drug concentration response relationships in normal volunteers after oral administration of losartan, an angiotensin II receptor antagonist. *Clin Pharmacol Ther* 1992; 51:513–521.

8. Li ZH, Bains JS, Ferguson AV. Functional evidence that the angiotensin antagonist losartan crosses the blood-brain barrier in the rat. *Brain Res Bull* 1993; 30:33–39.

9. Buj JD, Kimura B, Phillips MI. Losartan potassium, a non peptide antagonist of angiotensin II, chronically administered p.o. does not readily cross the blood brain barrier. *Eur J Pharmacol* 1992; 219:147–151.

10. Stevenson KM, Gibson KJ, Lumbers ER, et al. Comparison of the transplacental transfer of enalapril, captopril and losartan in sheep. *Br J Pharmacol* 1995; 114:1495–1501.

11. Goa KL, Wagstaff AJ. Losartan potassium: a review of its pharmacology and clinical efficacy in the management of hypertension. *Drugs* 1996; (in press).

12. Sica DA, Lo M-W, Shaw WC, et al. The pharmacokinetics of losartan in renal insufficiency. *J Hypertens* 1995: 13 (Suppl 1):S49–S52.

13. Chiu AT, McCall DE, Aldrich PE, et al. [3H]DUP 753, a highly potent and specific radioligand for the angiotensin II-I receptor subtype. *Biochem Biophys Res Commun* 1990; 172;1195–1202.

14. Abdelrahman A, Pang CCY. Competitive antagonism of pressor responses to angiotensin-II and angiotensin-III by the angiotensin-II 1 receptor ligand losartan. *Can J Physiol Pharmacol* 1992; 70:716–719.

15. Wong PC, Price WA, Chiu AT, et al. Nonpeptide angiotensin II receptor antagonists. VIII. Characterization of functional antagonism displayed by DuP 753, an orally active antihypertensive agent. *J Pharmacol Exp Ther* 1990; 252:719-725.

16. Cockcroft JR, Sciberras DG, Goldberg MR. Comparison of angiotensin-converting enzyme inhibition with angiotensin II receptor antagonism in human forearm. *J Cardiovasc Pharmacol* 1993; 22:579–584.

17. Christen Y, Waeber B, Nussberger J. Dose-response relationship following oral administration of DuP 753 to normal humans. *Am J Hypertens* 1991; 4(Suppl):350–353.

18. Gottlieb SS, Dickstein K, Fleck E, et al. Hemodynamic and neurohormonal effects of the angiotensin II antagonist losartan in patients with congestive heart failure. *Circulation* 1993; 88:1602–1609.

19. Dickstein K, Chang P, Willenheimer R, et al. Comparison of the effects of losartan and enalapril on clinical status and exercise performance in patients with moderate or severe chronic heart failure. *J Am Coll Cardiol* 1995; 26:438–445.

20. Crozier I, Ikram H, Awan N, et al. Losartan in heart failure. Hemodynamic effects and tolerability. Losartan Hemodynamic Study Group. *Circulation* 1995; 91:691–697.

21. Stapff M, Dueck KD, Richard F, et al. Evaluation of the antihy-

pertensive efficacy of losartan, an angiotensin II antagonist, compared to captopril using 24th ABPM [abstract no. 806]. Seventh European Meeting on Hypertension, 1995:183.

22. Brunier M, Rutschmann B, Nussberger J, et al. Salt-dependent renal effects of an angiotensin II antagonist in healthy subjects. *Hypertension* 1993; 22:339–347.

23. Doig JK, MacFadyen RJ, Sweet CS. Dose-ranging study of the angiotensin type I receptor antagonist losartan (DuP753/MK954), in salt-depleted normal man. *J Cardiovasc Pharmacol* 1993; 21:732–738.

24. Grossman E, Peleg E, Carroll J, et al. Hemodynamic and humoral effects of the angiotensin II antagonist losartan in essential hypertension. *Am J Hypertens* 1994; 7:1041–1014.

25. Tsunoda K, Abe K, Hagino T, et al. Hypotensive effect of losartan, a nonpeptide angiotensin II receptor antagonist, in essential hypertension. *Am J Hypertens* 1993; 6:28–32.

26. Fauvel JP, Laville M, Maakel N, et al. Effects of losartan on renal hemodynamic parameters in hypertensives [abstract]. *J Hypertens* 1994; 12(Suppl 3):93.

27. Nakashima M, Uematsu T, Kosuge K. Pilot study of the uricosuric effect of DuP-753, a new angiotensin II receptor antagonist, in healthy subjects. *Eur J Clin Pharmacol* 1992; 42:333–335.

28. van den Meiracker AH, Admiraal PJJ, Janssen JA, et al. Hemodynamic and biochemical effects of the AT1 receptor antagonist iresartan in hypertension. *Hypertension* 1995; 25:22–29.

29. Shaw W, Keane W, Sica D, et al. Safety and antihypertensive effects of losartan (MK-954; DUP753), a new angiotensin II receptor antagonist, in patients with hypertension and renal disease [abstract]. *Clin Pharmacol Ther* 1993; 53:140.

30. Gansevoort RT, de Zeeuw D, Shahinfar S, et al. Effects of the angiotensin II antagonist losartan in hypertensive patients with renal disease. *J Hypertens* 1994; 12 (Suppl 2):37–42.

31. Chan JCN, Critchley JAJH, Cockram CS, et al. Antihypertensive and anti-albuminuric effects of losartan potassium and felodipine-ER in elderly hypertensive Chinese with/without NIDDM [abstract]. *J Hypertens* 1994; 12 (Suppl 3):94.

32. Moan A, Hoieggen A, Eide I. Metabolic effects of antihypertensive treatment with the angiotensin II receptor antagonist losartan [abstract no. 551]. Seventh European Meeting on *Hypertension*, 1995; 126.

33. Sami H, Laurel C, Anderson PW. Effects of losartan treatment in hypertensive patients [abstract]. *J Invest Med* 1995; 43 (Suppl 1):199A.

34. de Zeeuw D, Gansevoort RT, Dullaart RPF, et al. Angiotensin II antagonism improves the lipoprotein profile in patients with nephrotic syndrome. *J Hypertens* 1995; 13 (Suppl 1):S53-S58.

35. Moan A, Risanger T, Eide I. The effect of angiotensin II receptor blockade on insulin sensitivity and sympathetic nervous system activity in primary hypertension. *Blood Press* 1994; 3:185–188.

36. Goldberg MR, Tanaka W, Barchowsky A, et al. Effects of losartan on blood pressure, plasma renin activity, and angiotensin II in volunteers. *Hypertension* 1993; 21:704–713.

37. Goldberg MR, Bradstreet TE, McWilliams EJ, et al. Biochemical effects of losartan, a nonpeptide angiotensin II receptor antagonist, on the renin-angiotensin-aldosterone system in hypertensive patients. *Hypertension* 1995; 25:37–46.

38. Ashino K, Gotoh E, Sumita S-I, et al. Efficacy of an angiotensin receptor antagonist, TCV-116, on sympathetic nerve activity in patients with essential hypertension. *Blood Press* 1994; 3(Suppl 5):122–129.

Rationale for Combined Therapy by β-Blockers and Calcium Antagonists

Mechanism

These two types of drugs both act hemodynamically: the β-blockers at least in part through reduction in cardiac output and the calcium antagonists by peripheral vasodilation. These mechanisms are complementary.

Side Effects

In general, combination therapy allows lower doses of each agent to be used, to achieve the same degree of blood pressure reduction. This means that combination therapy when used for patients with mild to moderate hypertension

TABLE 7-1. Comparative Contraindications of Verapamil, Diltiazem, Nifedipine, and of β-Adrenergic Blocking Agents

Contraindications	Verapamil	Diltiazem	Nifedipine (all DHPs)	Beta-Blockade
Absolute				
Sinus bradycardia	0/+	0/+	0	++
Sick sinus syndrome	++	+	0	++
AV conduction defects	++	++	0	++
Asthma	0	0	0	+++
Bronchospasm	0	0	0	++
Heart failure	++	++	++	0 or +
Hypotension	+	+	++	+
Coronary artery spasm	0	0	0	+
Raynaud's and active peripheral vascular disease	0	0	0	+
Severe aortic stenosis	+	+	++	+
Obstructive cardiomyopathy	0/+	0/+	++	+ (Indicated)*
Relative				
Insulin resistance	0	0	0	Care
Adverse blood lipid profile	0	0	0	Care
Quinidine therapy	Care	Care	Care**	Care
Disopyramide therapy	Care	Care	0	Care
Unstable angina	0	0	++	0
Postinfarct protection	Indicated (no LVF)	0 (no LVF)	++	Indicated

*Indicated means judged suitable for use by author (LH Opie), not necessarily FDA approved.
** Nifedipine depresses blood quinidine levels with rebound nifedipine withdrawal.
+++ = absolutely contraindicated; ++ = strongly contraindicated; + = relative contraindication; 0 = not contraindicated; AV = atrioventricular; LVF = left ventricular failure; DHP = dihydropyridine.

39. Graman AH, Arcuri KE, Goldberg AI, et al. A randomized, placebo-controlled, double-blind, parallel study of various doses of losartan potassium compared with enalapril maleate in patients with essential hypertension. *Hypertension* 1995; 25:1345–1350.

40. Weber MA, Byyny RL, Pratt JH, et al. Blood pressure effects of the angiotensin II receptor blocker, losartan. *Arch Intern Med* 1995; 155:405–411.

41. Dahlöf B, Keller SE, Makris L, et al. Efficacy and tolerability of losartan potassium and atenolol in patients with mild to moderate essential hypertension. *Am J Hypertens* 1995; 8:578–583.

42. Lappe JT, Nelson EB, Critchley JAJH, et al. Efficacy and tolerability of losartan potassium (MK-954, DuP 753), compared to felodipine ER in elderly hypertensive patients [abstract]. *J Hypertens* 1994; 12(Suppl 3):80.

43. Kjeldsen SE, Moan A, Sweet CS, et al. Treatment with the angiotensin II receptor antagonist losartan in 180 patients with severe hypertension [abstract]. *Am J Hypertens* 1994; 7(Part 2):33A.

44. Fletcher AE, Palmer AJ, Bulpitt CJ. Cough with angiotensin converting enzyme inhibitors: how much of a problem? *J Hypertens* 1994; 12(Suppl 2): S43–S47.

45. Lacourciere Y, Brunner H, Irwin R, et al. Effects of modulators of the renin-angiotensin-aldosterone system on cough. *J Hypertens* 1994; 12:1387–1393.

46. Goldberg AI, Dunlay MC, Sweet CS. Safety and tolerability of losartan potassium, an angiotensin II receptor antagonist, compared with hydrochlorothiazide, atenolol, felodipine ER, and angiotensin-converting enzyme inhibitors for the treatment of systemic hypertension. *Am J Cardiol* 1995; 75:793–795.

47. Acker CG, Greenberg A. Angioedema induced by the angiotensin II blocker losartan. *N Engl J Med* 1995; 333:1572.

48. Ogihara T, Arakawa K, Iimura O, et al. Open clinical studies on a new angiotensin II receptor antagonist, TCV 116. *J Hypertens* 1994; 12(Suppl 9):S35–S38.

49. Nagano M, Higaki J, Mikami H, Ogihara T. Role of the renin-angiotensin system in hypertension in the elderly. *Blood Press* 1994; 3(Suppl 5):130–133.

50. MacKay JH, Arcuri KE, Goldberg AI, et al. Losartan and low-dose hydrochlorothiazide in patients with essential hypertension. *Arch Intern Med* 1996; 156:278–285.

51. Schoenberger JA for the Losartan Research Group. Losartan with hydrochlorothiazide in the treatment of hypertension. *J Hypertens* 1995; 13(Suppl 1):S43–S47.

52. Soffer BA, Wright Jr JT, Pratt JH, et al. Effects of losartan on a background of hydrochlorothiazide in patients with hypertension. *Hypertension* 1995; 26:112–117.

53. Simpson RL, Morlin C, Toh J, et al. Efficacy and safety of losartan combined with hydrochlorothiazide in patients with mild to severe hypertension [abstract]. *Am J Hypertens* 1994; 7(Part 2):37A.

54. Velivis M, Dai XC, Goldberg AL, et al. Safety and efficacy of losartan potassium/hydrochlorothiazide combination tablet in patients with severe hypertension [abstract]. *Am J Hypertens* 1995; 8(Part 2):192.

55. Wexler RR, Greenlee WJ, Irvin JD, et al. Non-peptide angiotensin II receptor antagonists: the next generation in antihypertensive therapy. *J Med Chem* 1996;39:625–656.

CHAPTER 6

Combination Therapy of Calcium Channel Antagonists and Diuretics

Matthew R. Weir

Long-term clinical experience with diuretics has demonstrated their ability to lower blood pressure as well as reduce cardiovascular-related morbidity and mortality (1–3). They have been considered a baseline therapy for mild to moderate hypertension for decades. However, recent concerns about higher doses of diuretics on carbohydrate, lipid, and electrolyte metabolism have raised questions about safety (4–7). Consequently, research efforts have focused on the utility of combining lower doses of diuretics with other antihypertensive therapies in order to see if the use of one agent would counteract deleterious effects of another agent, and whether the drug mechanisms of action (which could be different) would therefore be additive. Additionally, it was hoped that lower dose regimens of both agents might provide efficacy and yet avoid individual toxicities that could be associated with titration to higher doses. Theoretically, the choice of an agent that would have additive blood pressure-lowering effects in combination with a diuretic would be particularly advantageous in hypertensive subjects with a lower renin, more salt-sensitive physiology, since these patients may not respond sufficiently to a single-agent nondiuretic therapy.

The purpose of this chapter is to describe the antihypertensive actions of diuretics and calcium channel antagonists in combination. The first section of the chapter will discuss the mechanism of action of the two classes of drugs to try to determine whether these actions may prove to be complementary or antagonistic. Subsequent discussion will focus on the controversy in the literature concerning whether or not diuretics and calcium channel antagonists have additive antihypertensive properties. A discussion about confounding variables in the studies as well as statistical design will limit the number of interpretable studies to address this question. Later sections in the chapter will focus on the types of study designs used and whether one sees similar effects if a diuretic is added to a patient not responding to a calcium channel antagonist or, vice versa, whether a calcium channel antagonist is added to a patient not responding to a diuretic. The impact of combining diuretic therapy with nondihydropyridine as well as dihydropyridine calcium channel antagonists will be discussed, as there is evidence in the literature of possible differences between the two. The chapter will conclude with a brief review of the studies that do provide proper methodology and sufficient statistical power to provide satisfactory answers as to whether or not these two classes of drugs do possess additive antihypertensive properties.

MECHANISMS OF ACTION

Considerable investigation has focused on the antihypertensive properties of diuretics and calcium channel antagonists. Despite much investigation, certain controversies about the mechanism of action of these drugs remain unsolved.

It is well known that thiazide diuretics induce natriuresis both acutely and with long-term administration (8–12), which may, in part, explain some of their antihypertensive properties. However, there is also evidence to suggest that greater dietary salt intake offsets the antihypertensive properties of diuretics, whereas reduced dietary salt enhances antihypertensive efficacy (13–17). Consequently, the antihypertensive properties of diuretics may well depend on the patients' dietary salt consumption despite the fact that there are conflicting studies as to the magnitude of this effect and whether it even exists, particularly at much lower dietary salt intake (18–20).

Other investigators suggest that diuretics lower blood pressure through mechanisms other than natriuresis. First, thiazides directly inhibit contraction of vascular smooth muscle (21). Second, thiazide diuretics will reduce blood pressure in patients with severe renal dysfunction (22), although others have demonstrated that dialysis patients do not exhibit a decrease in blood pressure when treated with thiazide diuretics (23). Third, thiazide diuretics may induce adrenergic hyposensitivity during long-term therapy (24). Fourth, blood pressure did not increase in thiazide-treated subjects during a high-salt diet despite despite a net-positive sodium balance (25). However, as previously mentioned, there is some controversy in this regard (13–17). Overall, these observations suggest that there may be nonrenal blood pressure-lowering effects of thiazide diuretics.

In summary, it appears that thiazide diuretics exert antihypertensive effects due to both mild natriuresis and diuretic-independent activities, perhaps through relaxation of vascular smooth muscle.

Calcium channel antagonists, like diuretics, also reduce blood pressure through natriuretic activities (26–35) and through specific effects on relaxing vascular smooth muscle (36). Intracellular calcium uptake is the major transducing signal whereby cell membrane stimulation results in cell activation. Consequently, pharmacological antagonism of cellular calcium uptake results in the inhibition of vascular smooth muscle contraction or induces vasorelaxation. In addition to vasodilatory effects, calcium channel antagonists also possess both acute and chronic natriuretic actions (26–35). It has been theorized that the mechanisms of natriuresis are in part hemodynamic, related to increased renal blood flow (30), and also may be related to specific antagonism of salt and water reabsorption in both the proximal and distal tubule of the nephron (26–29, 31). The relative potency of these two different antihypertensive properties of calcium channel antagonists has not been well studied.

One might theorize that since these two classes of drugs work in a similar fashion in reducing vascular tone and mild natriuretic effects, they might not be complementary in their ability to reduce systemic arterial pressure. However, there are some interesting clinical observations in response to changes in dietary salt that suggest that they may possess somewhat different antihypertensive properties. Although changing dietary salt intake may affect the antihypertensive effects of thiazide diuretics, higher salt intake does not offset the antihypertensive effects of calcium channel antagonists and there is no evidence to suggest that reduced dietary salt intake potentiates their antihypertensive activity (25, 33, 37, 38). There is also clinical evidence to suggest that calcium channel antagonists augment the diuretic actions of the loop diuretic bumetanide (39). Consequently, there are sufficient differences between the drugs in their relationship to dietary salt to warrant exploration as to whether they have additive or synergistic antihypertensive properties.

Clinical Trials

Unfortunately, clinical trials that evaluate blood pressure responses to combination therapy are especially prone to major errors of interpretation. This is particularly true as one starts to review the literature addressing the effects of diuretic-calcium channel antagonist combinations (40–43). Most clinical trials of combination therapy for hypertension have typically compared the effect of a single agent that has been titrated to a fixed level, usually in a situation where satisfactory blood pressure reduction has not occurred. This design answers the question as to whether a drug exhibits an additive effect in a nonresponding population; however, it does not address issues of complementary effects of the drugs across the full dosing range of each. A randomized factorial design that incorporates placebo and several doses of each of the test drugs will permit a full array of complementary effects to be demonstrated with each of the potential combinations, as well as permit an unbiased selection of the most effective combination of the two drugs (44). Crossover design trials with Latin square design may also provide satisfactory answers as long as there are sufficient patient numbers to provide adequate statistical power (45, 46). As with the factorial design trials, it is necessary to incorporate placebo in order to subtract out placebo responses.

Other issues of concern in interpreting combination clinical trials have to do with the definition of goal blood pressure reduction. With single drugs, reduction of systolic-diastolic blood pressure of 10/5 mmHg has been reported

(47). With combination therapy, Morgan and Anderson (46) have suggested that a reduction of systolic-diastolic blood pressure of 5/3 mmHg is significant. Which interpretation is appropriate? Similarly, the number of patients in each of the clinical trials needs to be carefully assessed along with the severity of their blood pressure, age, race, gender, and body habitus. In addition, dietary salt consumption may also play a role in either offsetting or augmenting the antihypertensive activities of diuretics. Needless to say, this could be a confounding variable.

In clinical trials looking for complementary activities of two drugs, the pharmacology of the drugs being studied is critical for the proper interpretation of the results. One may see additivity with lower doses of drugs in combination, whereas it may not be evident when much higher doses of a single agent are used. Similarly, some immediate-release calcium channel antagonists are short acting. Assessing antihypertensive additivity beyond the trough effect may miss the effect of one drug and demonstrate only the activity of the other drug. Similarly, at peak effect, the effect of one drug may overwhelm that of the other. With these concerns in mind, the subsequent discussion will focus on clinical trials evaluating blood pressure responses with the combination of diuretics and calcium channel antagonists.

References were sought from a Medline search of English language documents from 1966 to 1995 based on the search items *diuretic, calcium channel antagonist, hypertension,* and *human* to identify pertinent literature including review articles and editorials. Citations within each retrieved article were also searched for additional references. This comprehensive list was then limited to human clinical studies that evaluated the antihypertensive effects of diuretics and calcium channel antagonists.

As illustrated in Table 6-1, eight articles were identified that assessed the effects of diuretic therapy being added to patients whose blood pressure did not completely normalize with calcium channel antagonist therapy (47–54). These studies included both nondihydropyridine and dihydropyridine calcium channel antagonists. Five out of the eight studies demonstrated a complementary effect of different types of diuretics being added to calcium channel antagonists. Wicker and colleagues (47) in a small study demonstrated that the

TABLE 6-1. CLINICAL TRIALS OF DIURETICS ADDED TO PATIENTS NOT RESPONDING TO CALCIUM CHANNEL ANTAGONISTS

Author (Reference)	Calcium Channel Antagonist	Diuretic
Wicker et al., 1986 (47)	Verapamil	Althiazide, spironolactone
Frishman et al., 1987 (49)	Diltiazem	Mefruside
Massie et al., 1987 (50)	Diltiazem	Hydrochlorothiazide
Poulter et al., 1987 (51)	Nifedipine	Mefruside
Nicholson et al., 1989 (52)	Verapamil	Hydrochlorothiazide
Cappuccio et al., 1991 (53)	Amlodipine	Bendroflumethiazide
Franklin et al., 1996 (54)	Verapamil	Hydrochlorothiazide

combination of althiazide and spironolactone facilitated blood pressure reduction in verapamil nonresponders. Frishman and associates (48) showed that hydrochlorothiazide caused a further blood pressure reduction in verapamil-treated patients. However, this study was conducted with an open-label design. Massie and colleagues (50) demonstrated that hydrochlorothiazide facilitated blood pressure reduction in diltiazem nonresponders, whereas Poulter and associates (51) similarly found that mefruside promoted blood pressure reduction in nifedipine-treated but nonresponding patients (N = 17, supine systolic-diastolic blood pressure reduction of –8.5/–4.5 mmHg). More recently, Franklin and coworkers (54) reported that when nonresponders to 240 mg of verapamil (slow release) were treated with indapamide 2.5 mg daily, the blood pressure reduction when adding indapamide (systolic-diastolic blood pressure reduction of –8.6/–3.0 mmHg) was similar to that observed with the increase in verapamil to 480 mg (–7.6/–3.9 mmHg).

The three studies that demonstrated no benefit were small in size. The study of Schulte and colleagues (49), involving 36 patients, resulted in no additivity of mefruside when combined with diltiazem. Nicholson and associates (52) observed no benefit of adding 25 mg of hydrochlorothiazide to 13 verapamil nonresponders. Cappuccio and coworkers (53) did not see additional benefit when adding a diuretic to 12 patients with blood pressure nearly controlled by amlodipine.

Seven clinical trials were retrieved that evaluated whether calcium channel antagonists when added to diuretic nonresponders would facilitate blood pressure reduction (55–61) (Table 6-2). Six of these studies were conducted exclusively with dihydropyridines and all demonstrated that calcium channel antagonist supplementation to a diuretic nonresponder facilitated blood pressure reduction. These studies are limited by small study size with the exception of the papers by Schoenberger and colleagues (55), Carle and associates (58), Glasser and associates (60), and Zusman and coworkers (57). Schoenberger and colleagues (55) demonstrated that nitrendipine did facilitate blood pressure reduction in 41 patients not responding to 25 mg of hydrochlorothiazide compared to placebo. The blood pressure dropped from 148.6/96.0 ± 14.4/5.4 mmHg to 133.4/

TABLE 6-2. CLINICAL TRIALS OF CALCIUM CHANNEL ANTAGONISTS ADDED TO PATIENTS NOT RESPONDING TO DIURETICS

Author (Reference)	Diuretic	Calcium Channel Antagonist
Schoenberger et al., 1984 (55)	Hydrochlorothiazide	Nitrendipine
Hedner et al., 1986 (56)	Hydrochlorothiazide	Felodipine
Zusman et al., 1987 (57)	Hydrochlorothiazide	Nifedipine
Carle et al., 1988 (58)	Hydrochlorothiazide	Felodipine
Chrysant et al., 1989 (59)	Hydrochlorothiazide	Amlodipine
Glasser et al., 1989 (60)	Hydrochlorothiazide	Amlodipine
Opsahl et al., 1989 (61)	Hydrochlorothiazide	Nifedipine

85.4 ± 15.1/5.9 mmHg. Carle and associates (58) similarly demonstrated that felodipine, when added to 25 mg of hydrochlorothiazide nonresponders (N = 40), reduced diastolic blood pressure by 17 mmHg. Glasser and associates (60) added amlodipine to nonresponders to 50 mg of hydrochlorothiazide and demonstrated a significant blood pressure reduction of –14.2/–11.7 ± 2.3/1.0 mmHg (N = 46) compared to –4.5/–5.0 ± 2.7/1.2 mmHg (N = 45) with the diuretic alone. Similarly, Zusman and coworkers (57) demonstrated that nifedipine when added to hydrochlorothiazide did result in a further blood pressure reduction of –11.4/–10.5 mmHg over thiazide treatment alone (N = 50). Each of these four clinical trials involved at least 40 to 50 patients in each arm and were either comparative with another antihypertensive drug or placebo controlled.

Ten studies were identified that reported nonresponders to both calcium channel antagonists and diuretics having the opposite therapy added (61–71). These are outlined in Table 6-3. All of these studies suggested that the combination of the two therapies was more effective than the individual monotherapy. The study by Lacourciere (71) primarily focused on nonresponders to hydrochlorothiazide (12.5 mg) who had significantly improved, 24-hour ambulatory blood pressure control when amlodipine was added.

A total of seven clinical trials did not address additional therapy for nonresponders (44, 72–76) (Table 6-4). Marone and associates (72) conducted a crossover design trial using placebo, chlorthalidone, nifedipine, and the combination of chlorthalidone and nifedipine in 10 patients. They noted better blood pressure reduction with the combination as opposed to the individual monotherapies, as well as greater blood volume reduction with the diuretic-calcium channel antagonist combination compared to the calcium channel antagonist alone. Cappuccio and coworkers (73) conducted an unusual clinical trial where they assessed the ability of nifedipine, at peak effect (2 hours after dosing), to add to the antihypertensive effect of bendroflumethiazide. They ob-

TABLE 6-3. CLINICAL TRIALS EVALUATING NONRESPONDERS OF EITHER DIURETICS OR CALCIUM CHANNEL ANTAGONISTS HAVING OPPOSITE THERAPY ADDED

Author (Reference)	Diuretic	Calcium Channel Antagonist
Hallin et al., 1983 (62)	Bendroflumethiazide	Nifedipine
Massie et al., 1986 (63)	Hydrochlorothiazide	Nitredipine
Daniels and Opie, 1987 (64)	Hydrochlorothiazide, amiloride	Nisoldipine
Frishman et al., 1987 (65)	Hydrochlorothiazide	Diltiazem
Holzgreve et al., 1987 (66)	Hydrochlorothiazide	Verapamil
Zawada et al., 1987 (67)	Hydrochlorothiazide	Diltiazem
Benjamin et al., 1988 (68)	Bendroflumethiazide	Verapamil
Elliot et al., 1990 (69)	Numerous diuretics	Numerous calcium channel antagonists
Lacourciere et al., 1995 (71)	Hydrochlorothiazide	Amlodipine

TABLE 6.4. CLINICAL TRIALS UTILIZING FACTORIAL DESIGN
OR PARALLEL CROSSOVER STUDIES

Author (Reference)	Diuretic	Calcium Channel Antagonist
Marone et al., 1984 (72)	Chlorthalidone	Nifedipine
Cappuccio et al., 1986 (73)	Bendroflumethiazide	Nifedipine
Ferrara et al., 1987 (74)	Chlorthalidone	Nifedipine
MacGregor et al., 1987 (75)	Bendrofluazide	Nifedipine
Burris et al., 1990 (44)	Hydrochlorothiazide	Diltiazem
Salvetti et al., 1991 (77)	Chlorthalidone	Nifedipine
Weir et al., 1992 (78)	Hydrochlorothiazide	Diltiazem

served no greater effect at peak whether the patients were
on diuretic therapy or not. Ferrara and colleagues (74), in a
small study involving 14 patients, demonstrated that
chlorthalidone when added to nifedipine provided a better
antihypertensive effect compared to placebo.

MacGregor and associates (75, 76) performed studies
with a combination of nifedipine and bendrofluazide (Figure 6-1). When nifedipine was given to patients already
treated with the diuretic, there was an additional reduction
in blood pressure. However, when the diuretic was added to
the nifedipine-treated patients, there was no further reduction in blood pressure. These investigators theorized that
since nifedipine causes a long-term reduction in total body
sodium through its natriuretic effects, this could partially
explain the blunting of the antihypertensive effect of the diuretic when added to patients treated with nifedipine.

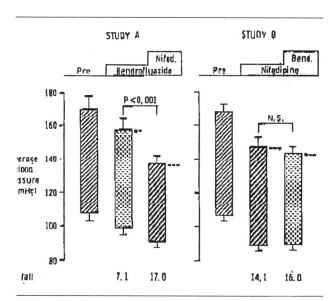

Figure 6-1. *Depicts difference in blood pressure reduction between adding
nifedipine (20 mg twice daily) to bendrofluazide therapy (5 mg daily) or
bendrofluazide (5 mg) to nifedipine therapy (20 mg twice daily) in 12 patients. The data illustrate average blood pressure after 1 month on each
therapy alone and after an additional month on combination therapy. *p<
.01, **p < .001 for the difference in blood pressures compared with pretreatment values. (Adapted with permission from MacGregor [76].)*

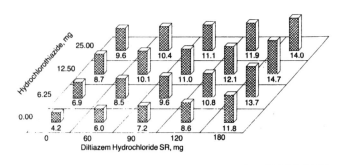

Figure 6-2. Mean supine diastolic blood pressure reduction (mmHg) in response to each therapy administered twice a day. SR = slow release. (Adapted with permission from Burris and associates [44].)

Salvetti and colleagues (77) randomized 66 patients to receive either nifedipine and placebo or chlorthalidone and placebo, or both chlorthalidone and nifedipine. They noted that there was no greater antihypertensive activity of the combination compared to the calcium channel antagonist alone. Unfortunately, despite using an adequate number of patients in a Latin square crossover study, they achieved almost normal blood pressure with nifedipine therapy alone, perhaps due to the inclusion of a number of borderline hypertensives. This may have explained the lack of additivity with the two drugs. More recently, Burris and associates (44) and Weir and colleagues (78) assessed the complementary activities of hydrochlorothiazide and diltiazem slow release [SR] using factorial design clinical trials. Burris and associates (44) in a double-blind, factorial design, placebo-controlled, parallel group multicenter study using placebo and three doses of hydrochlorothiazide (6.25, 12.5, 25 mg) and four doses of diltiazem SR (60, 90, 120, 180 mg twice daily), demonstrated that there was clear antihypertensive additivity between the two drugs (Figure 6-2). The blood pressure of the patients who received combination therapy was lower by an overall mean of 3 mmHg diastolic and 8 mmHg systolic versus the calcium channel antagonist used alone and 3.5 mmHg diastolic and 4 mmHg systolic versus diuretic used alone. In a follow-up study reported by Weir and colleagues (78), a randomized, placebo, parallel group study was conducted to delineate the optimal antihypertensive dosage of diltiazem SR and hydrochlorothiazide. Patients were randomized to receive either placebo (N = 75), hydrochlorothiazide (N = 76), diltiazem SR (N = 72), or the combination of diltiazem SR and hydrochlorothiazide (N = 75). A comparison of reduction in diastolic blood pressure between various evaluation periods during the study demonstrated a dose-response relationship for the combination therapy (diltiazem SR-hydrochlorothiazide 60/6.25, 90/6.25, 120/12.5 mg twice daily. The combination therapy exhibited enhanced efficacy relative to each monotherapy. Consequently, four of the six studies did demonstrate the complementary effects of these two different classes of drugs in reducing blood pressure despite the variety in numbers of patients utilized, study design, and the types of calcium channel antagonists and diuretics employed.

CONCLUSIONS

Overall, the majority of combination calcium channel antagonist-diuretic studies suffer from faulty trial design. Most commonly the studies suffer from lack of placebo controls, small numbers of patients studied, and insufficient power to ensure statistically significant reduction of blood pressure. Additionally, the majority of the studies have focused on the treatment of nonresponders without assessing a full-dose response range of each individual monotherapy with a factorial design. Those studies that did employ proper study design with sufficient numbers of patients demonstrated consistent antihypertensive additivity (with diltiazem and hydrochlorothiazide). Although similar studies have not been conducted with dihydropyridines or the nondihydropyridine verapamil, based on the existing data from well-done, parallel design clinical trials such as the results of Poulter and associates (51), Schoenberger and colleagues (55), Zusman and coworkers (57), and Glasser and associates (60), that similar, additive results on blood pressure reduction with these two classes of drugs would be observed. Although there may be theoretical grounds for believing that diuretics will not be complementary with calcium channel antagonists because inhibition of cellular calcium uptake by calcium channel antagonists will optimally attenuate vascular smooth muscle contraction and for believing that dietary salt variation does not affect the antihypertensive response to calcium channel antagonists, there is fairly consistent evidence in the literature reviewed herein to suggest that additive antihypertensive effects exist between these two classes of drugs.

REFERENCES

1. Veterans Administration Cooperative Study Group on Antihypertensive Agents. Effects of treatment on morbidity in hypertension: results in patients with diastolic blood pressure averaging 115 through 129 mmHg. *JAMA* 1967; 202:1028–1034.

2. Veterans Administration Cooperative Study Group on Antihypertensive Agents. Effects of treatment on morbidity in hypertension II: results in patients with diastolic blood pressure averaging 90 through 114 mmHg. *JAMA* 1970; 213:1143–1150.

3. SHEP Cooperative Research Group. Prevention of stroke by antihypertensive drug treatment in older persons with isolated systolic hypertension. *JAMA* 1991; 265:3255–3264.

4. Kasiske BL, Ma JZ, Kalil RSN, Louis TA. Effects of antihypertensive therapy on serum lipids. *Ann Intern Med* 1995; 122:133–141.

5. McKenney JL, Goodman R, Wright JT, et al. The effect of low-dose hydrochlorothiazide on blood pressure, serum potassium, and lipoproteins. *Pharmacotherapy* 1986; 6:179–184.

6. Harper R, Ennis CN, Sheridan B, et al. Effects of low dose versus conventional dose thiazide diuretics on insulin action in essential hypertension. *Br Med J* 1994; 309:226–230.

7. Curb JC, Maxwell MH, Schneider KA, et al. Adverse effects of anti-hypertensive medications in the hypertension detection and follow-up program. *Prog Cardiovasc Dis* 1986; 29(Suppl 1):73–88.

8. Freis ED, Wanko A, Wilson IM, Paris AE. Chlorothiazide in hypertensive and normotensive patients. *Ann N Y Acad Sci* 1958; 71:450–456.

9. Lauwers P, Conway J. Effect of long-term treatment with chlorothiazide on body fluids, serum electrolytes, and exchangeable sodium in hypertensive patients. *J Lab Clin Med* 1960; 56:401–408.

10. Wilson IM, Freis Ed. Relationship between plasma and extracellular fluid volume depletion and the antihypertensive effect of chlorothiazide. *Circulation* 1959; 20:1028–1036.

11. Freis ED, Wanko A, Schnaper HW, Frohlich ED. Mechanism of the altered blood pressure responsiveness produced by chlorothiazide. *J Clin Invest* 1960; 39: 1277–1281.

12. Freis ED, Reda DM, Materson BJ. Volume (weight) loss and blood pressure response following thiazide diuretics. *Hypertension* 1988; 12:244–250.

13. Beard TC, Gray WR, Cooke HM, Barge R. Randomized controlled trial of a no-added-sodium diet for mild hypertension. *Lancet* 1982; ii:455–463.

14. Winer BM. The antihypertensive mechanisms of salt depletion induced by hydrochlorothiazide. *Circulation* 1961; 24:788–796.

15. Johnson OD, Ruchelman H, Ford RV. Diuretics and hypertension: effect of sodium balance. *N Engl J Med* 1962; 267:336–338.

16. Fries ED, Wanko A, Wilson IM, Parrish AE. Treatment of essential hypertension with chlorothiazide. *J Am Med Assoc* 1958; 166:137–140.

17. Finnerty FA, Davidov M, Kakaviatos IV. Relation of sodium balance to arterial pressure during drug-induced natriuresis. *Circulation* 1968; 37:175–183.

18. Parijs J, Joossens JV, Van der Linder L, et al. Moderate sodium restriction and diuretics in the treatment of hypertension. *Am Heart J* 1973; 85:22–34.

19. Van Brummelen P, Schalekamp M, de Graeff J. Influence of sodium intake on hydrochlorothiazide-induced changes in blood pressure, serum electrolytes. *Acta Med Scand* 1978; 204:151–157.

20. Erwteman TM, Nagelkerke N, Lubsen J, et al. β-blockade, diuretics, and salt restriction for the management of mild hypertension: a randomized double blind trial. *Br Med J* 1984; 289:406–409.

21. Mironneau J, Savineau J-P, Mironneau C. Compared effects of indapamide, hydrochlorothiazide and chlorthalidone on electrical and mechanical activities in vascular smooth muscle. *Eur J Pharmacol* 1981; 75:109–113.

22. Jones B, Nanra RS. Double-blind trial of antihypertensive effect of chlorothiazide in severe renal failure. *Lancet* 1979; ii:1258–1260.

23. Bennett WM, McDonald WJ, Kuehnel E, et al. Do diuretics have antihypertensive properties independent of natriuresis? *Clin Pharmacol Ther* 1977; 22:499–504.

24. Middeke M, Remien J, Kirzinger S, Holzgreve H. Adrenergic hyposensitivity during long-term diuretic therapy a possible explanation for the antihypertensive effect of diuretics? *Eur J Pharmacol* 1985; 109:401–403.

25. Luft FC, Fineberg NS, Weinberger MH. Long-term effect of nifedipine and hydrochlorothiazide on blood pressure and sodium homeostasis at varying levels of salt intake in mildly hypertensive patients. *Am J Hypertension* 1991; 4:752–760.

26. Wallia R, Greenberg A, Puschett JB. Renal hemodynamic and tubular transport effects of nitrendipine. *J Lab Clin Med* 1985; 105:498–503.

27. DiBona GF, Sawin LL. Renal tubular site of action of felodipine. *J Pharmacol Exp Ther* 1984; 28:420–424.

29. Luft, FC, Weinberger MH. Calcium antagonists and renal sodium homeostasis. In: Epstein M. Loutzenhiser R, eds. *Calcium antagonist and the kidney*. Philadelphia: Hanley & Belfus, 1990: 203–212.

30. Loutzenhiser R, Epstein M. The renal hemodynamic effects of calcium antagonists. In: Epstein M, Loutzenhiser R, eds. *Calcium antagonists and the kidney*. Philadelphia: Hanley & Belfus, 1990: 33–74.

31. Hughes GS, Coward TD, Oexmann MJ, Conradi EC. Verapamil induced natriuretic and diuretic effects: dependency on sodium intake. *Clin Phamacol Ther* 1988; 44:400–407.

32. Zanchetti A, Leonetti G. Natriuretic effects of calcium antagonists. Clinical implications. *Drugs* 1990; 40 (Suppl 2):15–21.

33. Nicholson JP, Resnick LM, Laragh JH. The antihypertensive effect of verapamil at extremes of dietary sodium intake. *Ann Intern Med* 1987; 107:329–334.

34. Leonetti G, Rupoli L, Gradnik R, Zenchetti A. Effects of a low-sodium diet on antihypertensive natriuretic responses to acute administration of nifedipine. *J Hypertens* 1987; 5(Suppl 4):S57–S60.

35. Luft FC, Aronoff GR, Fineberg NS, Weinberger MH. Effects of oral calcium, potassium, digoxin and nifedipine on natriuresis in normal humans. *Am J Hypertens* 1989; 2:14–19.

36. Loutzenhiser R. Mechanisms of action of calcium antagonists. In: Epstein M, Loutzenhiser R, eds. *Calcium antagonists and the kidney*. Philadelphia: Hanley & Belfus, 1990: 1–22.

37. Nicholson JP, Resnick LM, DiFabio B, et al. Sodium restriction and the antihypertensive effect of nitrendipine [abstract]. *Clin Res* 1986; 34:404A.

38. Morgan T, Anderson A, Wilson D, et al. Paradoxical effect of sodium restriction on blood pressure in people on slow channel calcium blocking drugs. *Lancet* 1986; i:793.

39. Wilcox CS, Loon NR, Ameer B, Limacher MC. Renal and hemodynamic responses to bumetanide in hypertension: effects of nitrendipine. *Kidney Int* 1989; 36:719–725.

40. Weinberger MH. Additive effects of diuretics or sodium restriction with calcium channel blockers in the treatment of hypertension. *J Cardiovasc Pharmacol* 1988; Suppl 4:S72–S75.

41. MacGregor GD, Smith SJ, Sagnella GA. Why use angiotensin converting enzyme inhibitors to lower blood pressure? *J Cardiovasc Pharmacol* 1985; 7 (Suppl 4):S92–S97.

42. Weinberger MH. The relationship of sodium balance and concomitant diuretic therapy to blood pressure response with calcium channel entry blockers. *Am J Med* 1991; 90(Suppl 5A):15S–20S.

43. Sever PS, Poulter NR. Calcium antagonist and diuretics as combined therapy. *J Hypertens* 1987; 5(Suppl 4):S123–S126.

44. Burris JF, Weir MR, Oparil S, et al. An assessment of diltiazem and hydrochlorothiazide in hypertension. *JAMA* 1990; 263:1507–1512.

45. Sever PS, Poulter NR, Bulpitt CS. Double-blind crossover versus parallel groups in hypertension. *Am Heart J* 1989; 117:735.

46. Morgan TO, Anderson A. Hemodynamic comparisons of enalapril and felodipine and their combination. *Kidney Int* 1992; 41(Suppl 36):S78–S81.

47. Wicker P, Roudant R, Gosse P, Dallocchio M. Short- and long-term treatment of mild to moderate hypertension with verapamil. *Am J Cardiol* 1986; 57:83D–86D.

48. Frishman WH, Eisen G, Charlap S, Strom JA. Long-term safety and efficacy comparison of immediate-release and sustained-release oral verapamil in systemic hypertension. *J Clin Hypertens* 1987; 3:605–609.

49. Schulte KL, Meyer-Sabellek W, Rocker L, et al. Effects of diltiazem alone and combined with mefruside on cardiovascular response at rest and during exercise, carbohydrate metabolism and serum lipoprotein in patients with systemic hypertension. *Am J Cardiol* 1987; 60:826–831.

50. Massie B, MacCarthy P, Ramanathan KB, et al. Diltiazem and propranolol in mild to moderate essential hypertension as monotherapy or with hydrochlorothiazide. *Ann Intern Med* 1987; 107:150–157.

51. Poulter N, Thompson AV, Sever PS. A double-blind, placebo-controlled, crossover trial to investigate the additive hypotensive effect of a diuretic (mefruside) to that produced by nifedipine. *J Cardiovasc Pharmacol* 1987; Suppl 10:S53–S55.

52. Nicholson JP, Resnick LM, Laragh JH. Hydrochlorothiazide is not additive to verapamil in treating essential hypertension. *Arch Intern Med* 1989; 149:125–128.

53. Cappuccio FP, Markandu ND, Singer DRJ, et al. A double-blind crossover study of the effect of concomitant diuretic therapy in hypertensive patients treated with amlodipine. *Am J Hypertens* 1991; 4:297–302.

54. Franklin SS, Weir MR, Smith DHG, et al. Combination treatment with sustained release verapamil and indopamide in the treatment of mild-to-moderate hypertension. *Am J Therapeutics* 1996; (in press).

55. Schoenberger JA, Glasser SP, Ram CBS, et al. Comparison of nitrendippine combined with low-dose hydrochlorothiazide to hydrochlorothiazide alone in mild to moderate essential hypertension. *J Cardiovasc Pharmacol* 1984; 6:S1105–S1108.

56. Hedner T, Samuelsson O, Sjorgen E, Elmfeldt D. Treatment of essential hypertension with felodipine in combination with a diuretic. *Eur J Clin Pharmacol* 1986; 30:133–139.

57. Zusman A, Christensen O, Federman L, et al. Comparison of nifedipine and proprandolol used in combination with diuretics for the treatment of hypertension. *Am J Med* 1987; 82(Suppl 3B):37–41.

58. Carle WK, Latta D, Lees CTW, et al. A comparison of felodipine and propranolol as additions to hydrochlorothiazide in the treatment of hypertension. *Eur J Clin Pharmacol* 1988; 34:115118.

59. Chrysant SG, Chrysant C, Trus J, Hitchcock A. Antihypertensive effectiveness of amlodipine in combination with hydrochlorothiazide. *Am J Hypertens* 1989; 2:537–541.

60. Glasser SP, Chrysant SG, Graves J, et al. Safety and efficacy of amlodipine added to hydrochlorothiazide therapy in essential hypertension. *Am J Hypertens* 1989; 2:154–157.

61. Opsahl JA, Halstenson CE, Abraham PA. Antihypertensive and humoral effects of mifedipine in essential hypertension uncontrolled by hydrochlorothiazide alone. *Am J Hypertens* 1989; 2:828–833.

62. Hallin L, Andren L, Hansson L. Controlled trial of nifedipine and bendroflumethiazide in hypertension. *J Cardiovasc Pharmacol* 1983; 5(6):1083–1085.

63. Massie BM, Tabau JF, Szlachcic J, Vollmer C. Comparison and additivity of nitrendipine and hydrochlorothiazide in systemic hypertension. *Am J Cardiol* 1986; 38:16D–19D.

64. Daniels AR, Opie LH. Monotherapy with the calcium channel antagonist nisoldipine for systemic hypertension and comparison with diuretic drugs. *Am J Cardiol* 1987; 60:703–707.

65. Frishman WH, Zawada ET, Smith LK, et al. Comparison of hydrochlorothiazide and sustained-release diltiazem for mild-to-moderate systemic hypertension. *Am J Cardiol* 1987; 59:615–623.

66. Holzgreve H, Distler A, Michaelis J, et al. Verapamil versus hydrochlorothiazide in the treatment of hypertension: results of long-term double blind comparative trial. *BMJ* 1989: 299:881–886.

67. Zawada ET, Williams L, McClung DE, et al. Renal-metabolic consequences of antihypertensive therapy with diltiazem versus hydrochlorothiazide. *Miner Electrolyte Metab* 1987; 13:72–77.

68. Benjamin N, Phillips RJW, Robinson BF. Verapamil and bendrofluazide in the treatment of hypertension: a controlled study of effectiveness alone and in combination. *Eur J Clin Pharmacol* 1988; 34:249–253.

69. Elliott WJ, Polascik TB, Murphy WB. Equivalent antihypertensive effects of combination using diuretic and calcium antagonist compared with diuretic and ACE inhibitor. *J Hypertens* 1990; 4:717–723.

70. Boulet AP, Chockalingam A, Fodor JG, et al. Treatment of mild to moderate hypertension: comparison between a calcium channel blocker and a potassium sparing diuretic. *J Cardiovasc Pharmacol* 1991; 18(Suppl 9):S45–S50.

71. Lacourciere Y, Poivier L, Lefebvre J, et al. Antihypertensive effects of amlodipine and hydrochlorothiazide in elderly patients with ambulatory hypertension. *Am J Hypertens* 1995; 8:1154–1159.

72. Marone C, Luisoli S, Bomio F, et al. Pressor factors and cardiovascular pressor responsiveness after short-term antihypertensive therapy with calcium antagonist nifedipine alone or combined with a diuretic. *J Hypertens* 1984; 2(Suppl 3):449–452.

73. Cappuccio FP, Markandu ND, Rucker F, et al. Does a diuretic cause a further fall in blood pressure in hypertensive patients already on nifedipine? *J Clin Hypertens* 1986; 4:346–353.

74. Ferrara LA, Pasanisi F, Marotta T, et al. Calcium antagonists and thiazide diuretics in the treatment of hypertension. *J Cardiovasc Pharmacol* 1987; 10(Suppl 10):S136–S137.

75. MacGregor GA, Pevahouse JB, Cappuccio FP, Markandu ND. Nifedipine, sodium intake, diuretics, and sodium balance. *Am J Nephrol* 1987; 7(Suppl 1):44–48.

76. MacGregor GA. Nifedipine and hypertension: Roles of vasodilation and sodium balance. *Cardiovasc Drugs Ther* 1989; 3:295–301.

77. Salvetti A, Magagna A, Innocenti P, et al. The combination of chlorthalidone with nifedipine does not exert an additive antihypertensive effect in essential hypertensives: a crossover multicenter study. *J Cardiovasc Pharmacol* 1991; 17:332–335.

78. Weir MR, Weber MA, Punzi HA, et al. A dose escalation trial comparing the combination of diltiazem SR and hydrochlorothiazide with the monotherapies in patients with essential hypertension. *J Hum Hypertens* 1992; 6:133–138.

CHAPTER 7

Combination Therapy of Hypertension by β-Blockade with Calcium Antagonists

Lionel H. Opie

Although a combination of a β-blocking drug and a calcium antagonist is often used to control hypertension, there are few if any long-term studies concerning the overall effects of this combination. It undoubtedly reduces the blood pressure more than each agent singly. To understand the additive antihypertensive mechanisms first requires an analysis of the disparate mechanisms' effects of each of the two drug categories.

MECHANISMS OF ANTIHYPERTENSIVE ACTION OF β-BLOCKADE

Although β-blockers are among the drugs that are frequently recommended as first-line therapy, often as an alternative to diuretics, the exact mechanism of the antihypertensive effect is not yet fully understood. The antihypertensive mechanism appears to be multiple and may differ according to the β-blocker. For example, some β-blockers have vasodilating capacities by virtue of added intrinsic sympathomimetic activity (ISA) or as a result of inherent α-adrenergic blocking capacity.

In general, the use of standard β–blockers is followed by an initial rise in the total peripheral resistance, which is followed by a fallback to the starting line after some months (1, 2). In general, however, it is known that β–blockers without vasodilating capacity are, in the long run, nearly as effective antihypertensive agents as the others (3). Therefore, the basic mechanism whereby β-blockade has an antihypertensive effect cannot reside in vasodilation. Nonetheless, such vasoldilator capacity of certain agents helps to maintain the cardiac output better at a similar reduction of blood pressure (1).

The Basic Formula

It should be recalled that the basic formula is

$$BP = CO \times TPR$$

where BP = blood pressure, CO = cardiac output, and TPR = total peripheral resistance.

It is proposed that in young hypertensives a major cause of the blood pressure increase is the rise in the cardiac output, whereas in the elderly the major mechanism is the increase in the total peripheral resistance (4). Logically, β-blockers acting by reduction of cardiac output should be more effective in the younger patients and less in the older. This prediction appears to be true in the case of American black patients (5), in whom the β-blocker atenolol was virtually ineffective in the older age group, although relatively effective in the younger patients. Among the American white patients, however, the β-blocker was almost equally effective in younger and in older age groups.

This apparently surprising finding suggests that β-blockers act not only by reducing the cardiac output, but also by reducing the total peripheral resistance. Furthermore, their mechanism of action is such that they become relatively ineffective in elderly black patients. The most logical explanation for this is that black patients, as a group, have lower renin values and elderly patients also tend to have lower renin values. Therefore it would appear that the antirenin effect of β-blockers could explain these discrepancies. The kidney is known to release renin under several influences including β_1-adrenergic stimulation. Eventually, increased renin becomes translated into an increased total peripheral resistance.

Whether β-blockers are safe in white elderly patients is a different issue. The Medical Research Council study (6) shows that for equal degrees of blood pressure reduction, the diuretic group was able to reduce stroke and coronary events, whereas the β-blocker group (atenolol) only reduced stroke at equal reductions of blood pressure. Mortality apparently rose in the atenolol group. This surprising finding, which has been much criticized, does emphasize that there is an important difference between an outcome study and a blood pressure reduction study. In the case of combined β-blocker-calcium antagonist therapy for hypertension, there are no outcome studies.

When a vasodilatory β-blocker was compared with atenolol over 1 year in the younger hypertensives, there was no difference in the overall effects or side effects (3). There appear to be no such studies in the elderly in whom an effect on total peripheral resistance may be more important.

Thus, regarding antihypertensive mechanisms, they are multiple, including an early reduction in cardiac output, a later fall in total peripheral resistance, reduction of renin secretion, and, possibly, an added central effect. Some workers have proposed that a central effect may be important, even if the drug is only water soluble (like atenolol) because, presumably, it does penetrate the cerebrospinal fluid.

Vascular Effects of β-Blockers

Regarding the peripheral arterioles, there is early vasocon-striction followed by later normalization or sometimes even increased vasodilation. Regarding the brachial arteries, propanolol did not change compliance in the younger patients but the arteries became stiffer in the older patients (7). Here the evidence is that vasodilating β-blockers such as pindolol and dilevalol (no longer used) do have different effects (8). Another vasodilating β-blocker is celiprolol, again with vascular effects differing from atenolol. In the case of a β-blocker without vasodilating properties, the carotid artery pulse wave is relatively unaltered because of wave reflection from the undilated peripheral arterioles. Such differences may change in time, because the lessened blood pressure will also decrease the rate of ejection from the left ventricle into the aorta and thereby improve the mechanical properties of the aorta. Furthermore, late peripheral vasodilation will tend, with time, to diminish the reflected wave that travels from the peripheral arterioles to the aorta. Thus, the net effect of a β-blocker on the mechanical properties of the large arteries is initially not as beneficial in the case of a standard β-blocker as with a vasodilating β-blocker, but logic would say that in time these differences could become less. At present a speculation may be that the relative lack of effect of standard β-blockers on the large blood vessels may explain why atenolol in the elderly was not able to reduce hard end points such as coronary disease.

BASIC ANTIHYPERTENSIVE MECHANISMS OF CALCIUM ANTAGONISTS

Calcium antagonists are established vasodilators and act by inhibiting the L-type calcium channel of vascular smooth muscle. Thereby the total peripheral resistance is reduced. The blood pressure will fall. Furthermore, the reflected wave from the periphery back to the aorta will be diminished and aortic compliance will improve. In addition, in the case of the non dihydropyridine calcium antagonists, the reduction in heart rate and tendency to a negative inotropic effect may exert some antihypertensive effects (9). Because these drugs are not vascular selective, they tend to be less powerfully antihypertensive than the dihydropyridines such as nifedipine or amlodipine, and because of the vasodilation the negative inotropic effect is translated into only a modest fall in the cardiac output (9). Hence, even with the nondihydropyridines, peripheral vasodilation provides an important antihypertensive mechanism. A second example of the better antihypertensive capacity of the dihydropyridines versus the nondihydropyridines is the superiority of amlodipine versus verapamil (10). The mean doses used were amlodipine 9 mg daily and verapamil 160 mg twice daily. A word of warning though: Blood pressure reduction does not equal safety and we have, as yet, no outcome studies on calcium antagonists in hypertension.

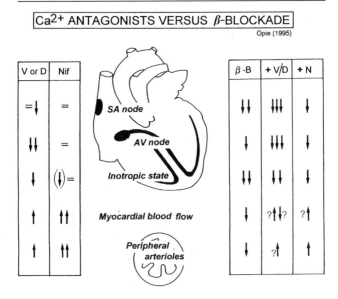

Figure 7-1. Comparative effects of Ca²⁺ antagonists and their combinations with β-blockade on the heart and circulation. Note that some of these effects are based on animal data, and extrapolation to man needs to be made with caution. V = verapamil; D = diltiazem; Nif = nifedipine; β–B = β-blockade; SA = sinoatrial; AV = atrioventricular. Figure © LH Opie.

Endothelial Effect

A recently described property of the calcium antagonist is to maintain endothelial integrity (11). While such endothelial protection is probably of major importance in patients with coronary disease, in the case of hypertension it is not yet sure that endothelial damage plays any significant role in the perpetuation or even in the initiation of the elevated blood pressure.

Neurohumoral Effects

By virtue of peripheral vasodilation, calcium antagonists as a group tend to increase renin and to promote adrenergic activation. These effects appear to be less in the case of the long-acting calcium antagonists because the short-acting variety causes intermittent vasodilation, particularly in the case of nifedipine. In the case of verapamil there is evidence that circulating noradrenaline is reduced and that renin is unaltered during long-term administration (12).

Metabolic Effects

There is some evidence that calcium antagonists improve insulin resistance and that in the particular case of verapamil, diabetic control might be better. Regarding blood lipid profiles, the calcium antagonists as a group are "lipid neutral."

should have fewer side effects. For example, a characteristic side effect of β-blockade is fatigue, whereas a typical side effect of calcium antagonism is peripheral edema. It might be anticipated, but it is not documented, that these side effects should be less during combination therapy.

Contraindications

An inspection of the contraindications (Table 7-1) shows that, in general, β-blockers combine better with the dihydropyridines than with the nondihydropyridines (verapamil and diltiazem). This theoretical difference, however, largely relates to the inhibitory effects of the nondihydropyridines on the sinus and atrioventricular node. In practice, the combination of β-blocker with nondihydropyridine calcium antagonist has often been made, provided due care is given to monitoring of the conduction on the electrocardiogram and provided that patients with cardiac complications are carefully assessed and followed up.

Safety

Although there are no long-term studies that allow comments on the safety of the combination β-blocker-calcium antagonist, in the Total Ischaemic Burden European Trial (TIBET) study (13) on patients with effort angina, combination therapy led to an increased blood pressure reduction (Table 7-2). These patients were not specifically hypertensive, but there is no reason to suppose that similar additive blood pressure reductions would not be found in hypertensives. Of interest, the TIBET study also compared the outcomes of the β-blocker and the calcium antagonist therapy, and found a similar incidence of hard end points (cardiac death, nonfatal myocardial infarction, unstable angina) and soft end points (coronary artery bypass surgery,

TABLE 7-2. CHANGES WITH TREATMENT IN HEART RATES AND BLOOD PRESSURES*

	Patients on Atenolol	Patients on Nifedipine	Patients on Combination
Number of patients	177	175	162
Sitting**			
HR	15.4 (0.08)	–2.9 (0.8)	13.5 (0.08)
SBP	12.9 (1.2)	12.5 (1.3)	20.6 (1.3)
DBP	7.3 (0.6)	6.7 (0.8)	11.0 (0.8)
Standing**			
HR	17.2 (0.8)	–3.7 (0.9)	15.6 (0.9)
SBP	12.8 (1.2)	13.6 (1.2)	20.4 (1.2)
DBP	7.5 (0.7)	6.5 (0.7)	11.4 (0.8)

*From TIBET Study, Dargie and colleagues (13), with permission of author and publisher. Patients with chronic effort angina, initial blood pressure not stated, but about 20% were hypertensive.
**Data are presented as mean (standard error) in mmHg. Figures represent mean fall in HR, SBP, and DBP; negative value represents an increase.
HR = heart rate; SBP = systolic blood pressure; DBP = diastolic blood pressure.

TABLE 7-3. EFFECTS OF DIFFERENT ANTIHYPERTENSIVE
AGENTS ON CORONARY RISK FACTORS

Clinical	Diuretic	Beta-Blocker	Calcium Blocker	ACE Inhibitors
Blood pressure	+	+	+	+
Serum total cholesterol	–			
Serum high-density lipoprotein cholesterol			–	
Left ventricular hypertrophy	±	+	+	+
Glucose intolerance	–	–		+
Hyperinsulinemia	–	–		+

ACE = angiotensin-converting enzyme; + = positive effect; – = negative effect.
(From Kaplan (17), with permission.)

coronary angioplasty, treatment failure) for an average follow-up of 2 years. This suggests that both agents are relatively safe in chronic stable angina, at least when compared with each other. Because this was not a large series, with a total number of 682 patients, this result does not settle the dispute about the possible adverse effects of calcium antagonists in relation to ischemic disease.

Logically, however, because part of the adverse effects of short-acting nifedipine are thought to be caused by reflex adrenergic activation, combination of a dihydropyridine with a β-blocker should improve safety.

Thus, even in situations in which short-acting nifedipine is no longer used, such as unstable angina and threatened myocardial infarction, the addition of a β-blocker conferred a therapeutic advantage and the combination was apparently safe (14, 15). It should be reemphasized that the use of nifedipine as the sole therapy in patients with threatened and acute myocardial infarction (AMI) is unsafe because mortality is increased (16).

Metabolic Effects

As can be seen from Table 7-3, the β-blockers and calcium antagonists have some different effects on lipids and glucose metabolism. Only β-blockers are thought to have adverse effects. The combination of a β-blocker plus a calcium antagonist should, theoretically, have few adverse metabolic effects because of the greater blood pressure reduction by the two different mechanisms. Thus, the expectation is that this combination should, for any given reduction of blood pressure, be more metabolically neutral than β-blockade alone.

Left Ventricular Hypertrophy

Both β-blockers and calcium antagonists have, in prospective trials, reduced LVH (18). Yet there is only indirect evidence that the combination is superior in this regard (18). Each of these two categories of drugs acts to reduce LVH by a different mechanism, so the combination should be superior.

PROJECTED OVERALL EFFECTS OF COMBINATION THERAPY WITH β-BLOCKERS AND CALCIUM ANTAGONISTS

Besides added effects on the blood pressure, such combination therapy can be expected to have a number of indirect benefits. Each of the major components of this therapy have been thought to have certain adverse effects or lack of beneficial effects in two groups of patients. In the single, prospective, placebo-controlled study conducted on the elderly (6), the β-blocker atenolol was not successful in reducing coronary disease or mortality. There are now a number of outcome trials underway in elderly hypertensives with calcium antagonists and it may be anticipated from their beneficial effects on aortic compliance that these agents will be better at reducing hard end points related to left ventricular function. On the other hand, calcium antagonists as a group have been questioned when used for patients with ischemic heart disease with reflex adrenergic activation as a possible explanation. Two studies in chronic effort angina suggest that calcium antagonists are as safe as β-blockers (13, 19). The overall safety of β-blockers in ischemic heart disease is not seriously in doubt, and β-blockade reduces adrenergic activation. Therefore the combination of β-blockers with a calcium antagonist should, theoretically, be safe and effectively hypotensive.

SUMMARY

At present, the arguments for the antihypertensive combination of a calcium antagonist with a β-blocker seem reasonable. In the absence of any randomized, controlled, prospective outcome studies in hypertension, there should correctly be an inherent reserve about extrapolating from the properties of each of these types of agents when given singly to their use in combination therapy. The combination is likely to control blood pressure when monotherapy fails. Its benefits are likely to exceed any disadvantages. From the practical point of view, it is easier to combine a dihydropyridine calcium antagonist than a nondihydropyridine with a β-blocker, so as to avoid any adverse effects on the sinoatrial or atrioventricular nodes.

REFERENCES

1. Opie LH. Role of vasodilation in the antihypertensive and antianginal effects of labetalol: implications for therapy of combined hypertension and angina. *Cardiovasc Drugs Ther* 1988; 2:369–376.

2. Man in't Veld A, van den Meiracker AH, Schalekamp MA. Do β–blockers really increase peripheral vascular resistance? Review of the literature and new observations under basal conditions. *Am J Hypertens* 1988; 1:91–96.

3. Ambrosioni E, Birkenhager W, De Leeuw P, et al. Comparison of a vasodilating β–blocker in a long-term treatment of hyperten-

sion: a European multicentre study. *J Hum Hypertens* 1989; 7:S266–S267.

4. Lund-Johansen P. Twenty-year follow up of hemodynamics in essential hypertension during rest and exercise. *Hypertension* 1991; 18:54–61.

5. Materson BJ, Reda DJ, Cushman WC, et al. Single-drug therapy for hypertension in men. A comparison of six antihypertensive agents with placebo. *N Engl J Med* 1993; 328:914–921.

6. MRC working party. Medical Research Council trial of treatment of hypertension in older adults: principal results. *BMJ* 1992; 304:405–412.

7. London GM, Laurent S, Safar ME. The autonomic nervous system and large conduit arteries. In: O'Rourke M, Safar M, Dzau V, eds. *Arterial vasodilation*. Philadelphia: Lea & Febiger, 1993; 167–179.

8. Kelly R. Haemodynamic benefit of vasodilating β–blockers in treatment of essential hypertension. In: O'Rourke M, Safar M, Dzau V, eds. *Arterial vasodilation*. Philadelphia: Lea & Febiger, 1993: 104–116.

9. Leenen FH, Fourney A. Comparison of the effects of amlodipine and diltiazem on 24-hour blood pressure, plasma catecholamines, and left ventricular mass. *Am J Hypertens* 1996; 78:203–207.

10. Lorimer AR, Smedsrud T, Walker P, Tyler MH. Comparison of amlodipine and verapamil in the treatment of mild to moderate hypertension. *J Cardiovasc Pharmacol* 1988; 2:S89–S93.

11. Frielingsdorf J, Seiler C, Kaufmann P, et al. Normalisation of abnormal coronary vasomotion by calcium antagonists in patients with hypertension. *Circulation* 1996; 93:1380–1387.

12. Kailasam MT, Parmer RJ, Cervenka JH, et al. Divergent effects of dihydropyridine and phenylalkylamine calcium channel antagonist classes on autonomic function in human hypertension. *Hypertension* 1995; 26:143–149.

13. TIBET, Dargie HJ, Ford I, et al. Total Ischaemic Burden European Trial (TIBET) effects of ischaemia and treatment with atenolol, nifedipine SR and their combination on outcome in patients with chronic stable angina. *Eur Heart J* 1996; 17:104–112.

14. HINT, Trial Holland Interuniversity Nifedipine/Metoprolol. Early treatment of unstable angina in the coronary care unit; a randomised, double-blind, placebo controlled comparison of recurrent ischaemia in patients treated with nifedipine or metoprolol or both. *Br Heart J* 1986; 56:400–413.

15. Muller J, Morrison J, Stone PH, et al. Nifedipine therapy for patients with threatened and acute myocardial infarction: a randomized, double-blind, placebo-controlled comparison. *Circulation* 1984; 69:740–747.

16. Muller JE, Turi ZG, Pearl DL, et al. Nifedipine and conventional therapy for unstable angina pectoris: a randomized, double-blind comparison. *Circulation* 1984; 69:728–739.

17. Kaplan NM. Combination therapy for systemic hypertension. *Am J Cardiol* 1995; 76:595–597.

18. Cruickshank JM, Lewis H, Moore V, Dodd C. Reversibility of left ventricular hypertrophy by differing types of antihypertensive therapy. *J Hum Hypertens* 1992; 6:85–90.

19. APSIS, Rehnqvist N, Hjemdahl P, et al. The angina prognosis study in Stockholm (APSIS). Effects of metoprolol vs. verapamil in patients with stable angina pectoris. *Eur Heart J 1996*; 17:76–81.

CHAPTER 8

Beta-Blockers and ACE Inhibitors

Gustav G. Belz

Beta-blockers (i.e., β-adrenoceptor antagonists) and ACE inhibitors are frequently considered to exert their antihypertensive effects mainly via the same mechanism (i.e., a suppression of the activity of the renin-angiotensin-aldosterone system). A combination of these two classes of drugs had therefore not entered the classical hypertension stepcare schemata. The arguments against this combination mainly arose from theoretical considerations, but in contrast several clinical studies have found the combination to be of clinical value. This discussion covers the underlying physiological and pharmacological bases for the action of these drugs and their combination, with special consideration to counterregulatory mechanisms.

THEORETICAL CONSIDERATIONS

Effects of β-Blockers on Blood Pressure

Although introduced for the treatment of hypertension almost three decades ago (1), the mechanisms of β-blocker antihypertensive action are not yet completely understood and there probably exist several mechanisms by which they influence blood pressure. The influence of the sympathetic nervous system on the regulation of blood pressure is presented schematically in Figure 8-1. Norepinephrine causes a rise in blood pressure via (i) β_1-adrenoceptor stimulation, leading to an increase in cardiac output and increased secretion of renin from the juxtaglomerular apparatus of the kidney (thereby starting the renin-angiotensin-aldosterone cascade), and (ii) direct vasoconstriction mediated by stimulation of the α_1-adrenoceptor (2).

In contrast to norepinephrine, epinephrine mediates a vasodilatation via the β_2-adrenoceptor. This mechanism, however, is only of minor relevance under resting conditions when norepinephrine is the main catecholamine. During isotonic exercise and in response to some pathophysiological conditions like hypoglycemia and myocardial infarction, liberation of epinephrine plays a more important role (3).

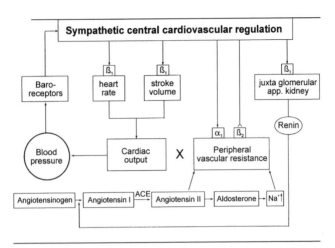

Figure 8-1. Sympathotonic central cardiovascular regulation. (Modified with permission from Palm [2].)

Since β_1-selective-blockers lower the blood pressure as well as or even better than nonselective β-blockers, the main mechanism of antihypertensive action must depend on the blockade of β_1-mediated effects of noradrenaline. Blood pressure can be described (hemodynamically) as the product of cardiac output and peripheral resistance. Cardiac output is a product of heart rate and stroke volume, and, via the drop in the heart rate, is reduced by β-blockers at least initially. In addition, when following β-blockers, the duration of diastole is lengthened and diastolic blood pressure decreases to a lower level before the next heartbeat (4). This "diastolic" effect can be considered to present an additional hemodynamic mechanism contributing to the lowering of blood pressure following β-blockade.

Since the α_1-adrenoceptors of the sympathetic system are not blocked, and especially since norepinephrine release is even intensified under β-blockade (5, 6), the peripheral vascular resistance increases (7) via stimulation of the α_1-adrenoceptors. This is visible as an increase in total peripheral resistance and may be considered to represent a counterregulatory attenuation of the blood pressure-lowering effect mediated by β_1-blockade (see Figure 8-1). Nonselective β-antagonists cause additional blockade of β_2-mediated vasodilating epinephrine effects and these substances are therefore characterized by a tendency to vasoconstrict, which may become clinically relevant (e.g., by cold extremities).

The blockade of the β_1-adrenoceptors at the juxtaglomerular apparatus leads to a reduction of renin secretion (6). Less angiotensin I and II are therefore produced from angiotensinogen and this results in an attenuation of the renin-angiotensin-aldosterone cascade.

In addition to these hemodynamic and humoral antihypertensive mechanisms of β-blockers, other mechanisms (e.g., central nervous system effects) have been proposed. An excellent overview on this topic is given by Cruickshank and Prichard (7).

Effects of ACE Inhibitors on Blood Pressure

Angiotensin II is formed from angiotensin I via ACE. It exerts its pressoric effects via at least two different mechanisms: (1) instantaneous, direct, strong arterial vasoconstriction, measurable as an increase in total peripheral resistance and consequently of blood pressure (8); and (2) slowly by sodium retention consequent to an increase of aldosterone secretion. An additional mechanism is the facilitation of norepinephrine release at the presynaptic receptor site (9, 10). ACE inhibitors inhibit the formation of angiotensin II and thereby exert a blood pressure-lowering effect. In addition, the accumulation of kinines, like bradykinin (since ACE is identical with kininase II), exert direct vasodilating and consequently blood pressure-lowering effects (11).

ACE inhibitors result in an intensified plasma renin release from the kidney due to the withdrawal of angiotensin II negative feedback and also to the drop in blood pressure. This leads to an accumulation of angiotensin I, which is hemodynamically inactive. This increase in plasma renin activity in animal experiments (cat) has been shown to be largely abolished by denervation of the kidney, suggesting a major role of the sympathetic nervous system (12). This observation also explains why plasma renin activity is lowered by β-adrenoceptor antagonists.

Despite almost complete blockade of ACE, the generation of angiotensin II will continue via chymase, which is not inhibited by ACE inhibitors. In addition one has to take into account the increased angiotensin I concentrations during the administration of ACE inhibitors, which are substrate for the chymase activity (13, 14). Angiotensin I, by conversion to angiotensin II, can bring about vasoconstriction. Therefore, even high doses of ACE inhibitors will not completely suppress angiotensin II production (15), resulting in an attenuation of the blood pressure-lowering effects of ACE inhibitors.

What Are the Theoretical Arguments—Contra and Pro—Combining β-Blockers and ACE Inhibitors?

Since at least a great proportion of the effects of β_1-blockade on hypertension is brought about by a blockade of the renin-angiotensin system, it seems to make little sense to add another drug acting mainly by the same mechanism (i.e., reduction of the amount of angiotensin II and aldosterone).

Conventional vasodilators (e.g., hydralazine, dihydropyridine derivatives, and other calcium antagonists) induce an intensive sympathetic stimulation mainly seen as a reflex tachycardia. These effects can be easily antagonized by β-blockers (16, 17). ACE inhibitors can be considered to act as vasodilators. They do not induce reflex tachycardia and in contrast exert some antisympathotonic effects (via withdrawal of angiotensin II-induced facilitation of noradrenaline release). Consequently there seems no need for additional beta-adrenoceptor blockade (18).

These *prima facie* convincing arguments do not take into account all aspects of the physiological and pharmacological mechanisms: There is no doubt that ACE inhibitors cannot prevent the formation of angiotensin II completely, as stated earlier. The strong rise in plasma renin activity following an ACE inhibitor should be blocked at least in part by coadministration of a β-blocker. The accumulation of angiotensin I should be markedly diminished. Thus, less substrate for any bypass transformation of angiotensin I to angiotensin II (e.g., by chymase activity) should be available and this should result in further reduced stimulation of the angiotensin II receptor. Conversely, the increase in peripheral resistance as seen after β-blockade alone should be attenuated when there is an additional lowering of the angiotensin II concentrations at the AT_1-receptors of the human smooth muscle by coadministration of the ACE inhibitor.

Another point is that though ACE inhibitors have some antisympathetic effects, these are only weak and insufficient to block stress- or exercise-induced sympatho-adrenergic blood pressure increases. The combination with a β-blocker could have the additional advantage of improved control of stress-induced increases in blood pressure.

In the following sections, the outcomes of studies dealing with the humoral, hemodynamic, and clinical effects of the combination of β-blockers and ACE inhibitors will be presented and discussed.

STUDIES ON THE HUMORAL INTERACTIONS BETWEEN β-BLOCKERS AND ACE INHIBITORS

In 1981 Staessen and colleagues (19) found that the increase in plasma renin activity and angiotensin I induced by captopril was significantly attenuated by coadministration of propranolol in hypertensive patients. Several other authors (20–22) confirmed the attenuation of the rise in plasma renin activity following captopril after the coadministration of propranolol. Pickering and associates (20) observed that the greatest reduction in urinary aldosterone excretion was produced by the two drugs in combination, suggesting that their synergistic effect was due to a more profound reduction in angiotensin II levels.

In a randomized, placebo-controlled, double-blind study in healthy volunteers, we evaluated the interaction between the nonselective β-blocker propranolol and the ACE inhibitor cilazapril (23) (Table 8-1).

Plasma renin activity was markedly increased 2 hours post cilazapril (factor ≈ 10, as compared with placebo). During the administration of propranolol alone, there was no significant effect on plasma renin activity. Following coadministration of both drugs, the ACE inhibitor-induced increase in plasma renin activity was markedly reduced (factor ≈ 3, as compared to cilazapril alone). The behavior of angiotensin I concentrations paralleled that of plasma renin activity and the ACE inhibitor-induced increase was markedly dampened by the coadministration of propranolol. Cilazapril alone induced only a small (≈ 10%) reduction of

TABLE 8-1. INFLUENCE OF A 1-WEEK ADMINISTRATION OF PLACEBO, CILAZAPRIL, PROPRANOLOL, AND THE COMBINATION OF CILAZAPRIL PLUS PROPRANOLOL ON PLASMA ENZYME AND HORMONE CONCENTRATIONS IN HEALTHY VOLUNTEERS

	Placebo	Cilazapril (2.5 mg/day)	Propranolol (120 mg/day)	Cilazapril 2.5 mg/day plus Propranolol 120 mg/day
Plasma renin activity ($ng \cdot ml^{-1} \cdot h^{-1}$)	1.6 (1.1)	17.9 (6.1)[xxx†††]	1.0 (0.4)[+++]	5.2 (7.0)[+]
Plasma angiotensin I ($pg \cdot ml^{-1}$)	112 (41)	699 (302)[xx††]	89 (23)[x++]	296 (326)[+]
Plasma angiotensin II ($pg \cdot ml^{-1}$)	34 (11)	30 (9)	32 (8)	25 (9)

*Mean +/− standard deviation. (Modified with permission from Belz and colleagues [23].)
Statistically significant differences: [x] vs. placebo, [+] vs. cilazapril, [†] vs. propranolol. One symbol, $p < .05$; two symbols, $p < .01$; three symbols, $p < .001$.

plasma angiotensin II concentrations, whereas there was no visible effect after propranolol alone. Following the coadministration of both drugs, angiotensin II concentrations decreased by about 30%. This result, though not having reached statistical significance in this study probably due to a small sample size, is in agreement with and confirms the findings on aldosterone (20).

A comparison of the results with plasma renin activity in these healthy volunteers and in hypertensive patients (Figure 8-2) revealed almost identical values for the two groups following placebo (24). The cilazapril-induced in-

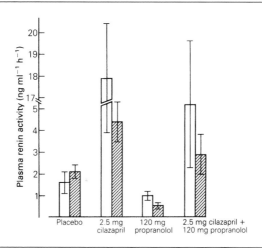

Figure 8-2. Influence of placebo, cilazapril 2.5 mg/day, propranolol 120 mg/day, and the combination thereof on plasma renin activity. Results (mean ± standard error mean of 2 hours after drug intake) compiled from a study in supine healthy volunteers (□, N = 6, treatment periods 1 week each) and sitting hypertensive patients (▨, N = 13, treatment periods with active drug 3 weeks each). (Reprinted with permission from Belz and colleagues [24].)

crease in plasma renin activity appeared more pronounced in healthy volunteers compared to hypertensive patients. Propranolol alone had no significant effect on plasma renin activity. Following the coadministration of both drugs, the cilazapril-induced increase in plasma renin activity was markedly reduced in both groups.

STUDIES ON THE HEMODYNAMIC INTERACTIONS BETWEEN β-BLOCKERS AND ACE INHIBITORS

Cardiac output and total peripheral resistance determine blood pressure (see Figure 8-1). Therefore, to obtain more insight into the mechanisms of action of drugs on blood pressure, one needs to see their influence on these basic variables.

Hemodynamic effects were evaluated in hypertensive patients noninvasively at rest and during isometric and isotonic stress, after a placebo run-in and after treatment periods of 3 weeks each with cilaz0april (2.5 mg/day), propranolol (120 mg/day), and their combination, respectively (25, 26). Both monotherapies had yielded significant and similar reductions in blood pressure, and the effect was more pronounced following treatment with the combination.

On cilazapril, heart rate was slightly reduced. On propranolol treatment, heart rate (as expected) decreased significantly. Combination therapy caused heart rate reductions similar to those observed during therapy with propranolol alone.

Cilazapril decreased total peripheral resistance and increased cardiac output at rest and during isometric exercise, whereas propranolol produced the opposite reactions. Combination therapy in comparison to placebo slightly decreased mean cardiac output as well as the total peripheral resistance. Thus, from the hemodynamic point of view, both cardiac output and total peripheral resistance were lowered following the combination of β-blocker and ACE inhibitor (Figures 8-3 and 8-4). Compared to the monotherapies, this resulted in a further blood pressure decrease.

Cardiopulmonary exercise testing in these hypertensive patients suggested that monotherapy with propranolol decreased the aerobic exercise capacity and exercise tolerance, while monotherapy with cilazapril improved it. When cilazapril and propranolol were coadministered, these effects were partially attenuated (for details see [26]).

STUDIES ON THE BLOOD PRESSURE-LOWERING EFFECT OF THE COMBINATION BETWEEN β-BLOCKERS AND ACE INHIBITORS

Studies in Healthy Volunteers

In a placebo-controlled, randomized, double-blind study in healthy volunteers we found identical decreases in systolic and diastolic blood pressures of 7 mmHg after treatment

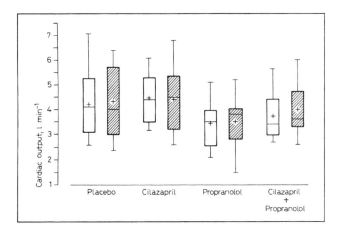

Figure 8-3. *Cardiac output sitting at rest (☐) and during isometric exercise (▨) 2 to 3 hours after the last drug intake sitting at rest and during isometric exercise (3-min. handgrip) after 2 weeks on placebo, 3 weeks on cilazapril, 3 weeks on propranolol, and 3 weeks on a combination of the two. Shown are the range, upper and lower quartile, median (-), and mean (+) of 17 patients. (Reprinted with permission from Erb and associates [26].)*

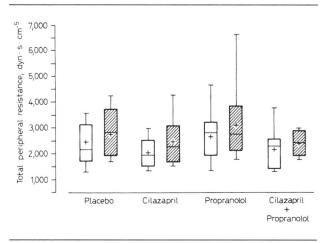

Figure 8-4. *Total peripheral resistance sitting at rest (☐) and during isometric exercise (▨) according to conditions described in Figure 8-3. (Reprinted with permission from Erb and associates [26].)*

with propranolol 120 mg/day (1 week) or cilazapril 2.5 mg/day (1 week) (with placebo there was no effect). The coadministration of both drugs reduced the diastolic blood pressure by about 18 mmHg and the effect was attained for a longer time period (Figure 8-5). These results in healthy volunteers were confirmed in other studies evaluating the interactions between ramipril (5 mg/day), propranolol (40 mg/day), and their combination (27); and between imidapril, bisoprolol, and their combination (data on file).

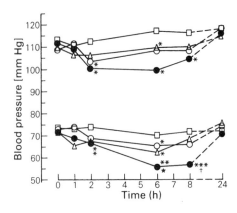

Figure 8-5. Blood pressure on the last day of a 1-week treatment period with placebo (□), propranolol 120 mg/day (△), cilazapril 2.5 mg/day (○), and propranolol 120 mg/day, plus cilazapril 2.5 mg/day (●). The mean values (N = 6) are shown. Statistical significances: ✱ vs. placebo, † = vs. propranolol; single symbol, p< .05; double symbols, p < .01; triple symbols, p < .001. (Reprinted with permission from Belz and colleagues [23].)

Studies in Hypertensive Patients

An earlier clinical paper from Staessen and colleagues (19) reported on hypertensive patients treated with captopril (200 mg three times a day) who were studied by adding propranolol (80 mg three times a day) or placebo in a crossover design. During monotherapy with captopril, diastolic blood pressure had remained elevated between 90 and 114 mmHg. The addition of propranolol produced a significant ($p < .01$) decrease in diastolic blood pressure of about 10 mmHg, accompanied by a drop in heart rate.

In a study by Pickering and associates (20), these results were confirmed and the authors found an average decrease in sitting diastolic blood pressure following captopril (average dose 350 mg daily) of 11 mmHg, propranolol (average dose 144 mg daily) of 9 mmHg, and by the combination of 17 mmHg. These authors had not only evaluated blood pressure at rest but also during physical exercise. They concluded that the cardiac output-decreasing effect of propranolol may be important during exercise (20), when the effects of the ACE inhibitors are limited (28).

When 12 hypertensive patients in a study by Mac-Gregor and colleagues (21) received propranolol (20 to 80 mg thrice daily) added to captopril (150 mg thrice daily) for 1 month, this did not appear to be a very effective combination. In contrast, treatment with the combination even resulted in somewhat higher supine blood pressure values when compared to captopril monotherapy.

The mild pressor effect of the coadministration of propranolol was considered analogous to the spurious reports of such an effect in hypertension with low renin status. As discussed earlier, these observations may be related to unopposed α-adrenoceptors and should be found with non-β_1-selective-blockers only.

In a study to assess blood pressure at rest and during ergometry (50 to 100 W), the effects of 100 mg of a β_1-selective-blocker, atenolol, 20 mg of enalapril, and a low-dose combination of 50 mg atenolol plus 10 mg enalapril were compared in 25 hypertensive patients (29). After 4 weeks of treatment, blood pressure at rest was identically lowered by the two monotherapies and the effect was somewhat more pronounced after treatment with the combination, though only half of the dose of each of the substances had been used. During exercise, enalapril reduced systolic blood pressure by 6.2%, whereas atenolol yielded 15.8% and the combination yielded 18.4%. Thus, the combination produced a significant supplementary antihypertensive effect although the dosages of the individual drugs were lower. In another study, the effect of the combination of enalapril with atenolol (30) had been found to be not fully additive compared to the two monotherapies.

In a double-blind study (31) the addition of a once-daily dose of either lisinopril (10 to 20 mg daily) or placebo to a pretreatment with atenolol was compared in 100 patients whose blood pressure was inadequately controlled by atenolol alone (50 mg daily). Blood pressures were taken at trough. The difference in favor of the ACE inhibitor was 7.1 mmHg compared to 5.4 mmHg with placebo ($p < .01$). The authors concluded that the addition of an ACE inhibitor to a pretreatment with a β-blocker produces a worthwhile decrease in blood pressure (31).

In contrast, Ferguson and colleagues (32) found no additive effect when testing single doses of captopril or propranolol, or their combination, on blood pressure at rest and during isometric and isotonic stress. The combination induced an effect similar to the effect obtained with the β-blocker alone.

We compared the antihypertensive effect of cilazapril (2.5 mg/day) and propranolol (120 mg/day) and their combination (25). Both monotherapies lowered diastolic blood pressure equally (average, –10 mmHg) and the combination lowered diastolic blood pressure significantly more (average –20 mmHg) (Figure 8-6). In these hypertensive patients (diastolic blood pressures on inclusion between 95 and 125 mmHg), a sitting diastolic blood pressure of ≤ 90 mmHg was achieved in 6 out of 17 patients with propranolol alone, in 8 out of 18 with cilazapril, and in 14 out of 17 with the combination. It could be of interest that the combination appeared to be better tolerated subjectively than the β-blocker alone. It should be stressed that the more pronounced effect of the combination was not due to a pharmacokinetic interaction of the drugs. Their plasma concentrations were almost identical with those of monotherapies (23).

In a study of the combination of metoprolol and ramipril, blood pressure was evaluated by 24-hour ambulatory blood pressure measurements (ABPM) (33). Twenty patients whose blood pressure was ineffectively controlled after 4 weeks of therapy with ramipril 2.5 mg/day received a combination of ramipril 2.5 mg and metoprolol 100 mg/day. After 4 weeks of treatment with the combination, 15 patients became normotensive and the percentage of el-

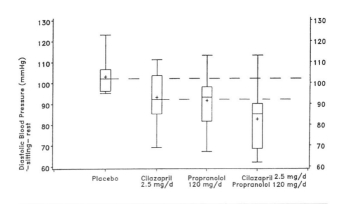

Figure 8-6. *Sitting diastolic blood pressure 2 hours after last drug intake at rest after 2 weeks on placebo, 3 weeks on cilazapril, 3 weeks on propranolol, and 3 weeks on a combination of the two drugs. The box-and-wisker-plots show the range, the upper and lower quartiles, the median (-), and the mean (+) of the 17 participating patients. For the sake of clarity, the median values for placebo and cilazapril are indicated by dashed lines. (Reprinted with permission from Belz and colleagues [25].)*

evated blood pressure values during the 24-hour ABPM was significantly reduced by the combination. The authors made an additional interesting observation: Whereas the peaks of systolic blood pressure exceeding 180 mmHg during ramipril alone amounted to 7% of the blood pressure registrations, these values decreased to 1% after the coadministration of metoprolol. The authors concluded that the combination should be especially useful in younger patients with increased sympathetic drive or in patients suffering from coronary heart disease (CHD) (33).

A Finnish group (34) evaluated the effects of adding to preexisting treatment with atenolol (50 mg/day), either the ACE inhibitor lisinopril (10 to 20 mg/day) or the diuretic hydrochlorothiazide (12.5 to 25 mg/day). In this double-blind, randomized study, the authors could not find any important difference between the combinations of the β-blocker with the thiazide diuretic or with the ACE inhibitor, neither in terms of efficacy nor of tolerability. Both combinations resulted in improved blood pressure control in comparison with atenolol alone.

A similar study has been published by Bursztyn and colleagues (35). One hundred twenty-seven patients whose blood pressure failed to normalize with atenolol monotherapy were evaluated for their response in blood pressure after addition of either benazepril (10 mg twice daily, increase after 1 week to 20 mg twice daily if necessary) or placebo. In the benazepril group 46% achieved an excellent or good response (i.e., diastolic blood pressure <90 mmHg or a decrease of >10 mmHg) in comparison with only 14% in the placebo group. The mean decreases in diastolic blood pressure at the end of the study were 5.6 mmHg in the benazepril and 3.7 mmHg in the placebo groups. Six of the patients in the ACE inhibitor group had an increase in blood pressure that offset the fall in the responders; therefore the difference in diastolic blood pressure response between the two groups was not statistically significant. However, the authors concluded that addition of an ACE inhibitor to the treatment regimen of patients whose blood pressure is inadequately controlled by a β-blocker can result in an additional decrease in diastolic blood pressure in almost half of the patients.

The Swedish lisinopril group study (36) comprised 340 hypertensive patients who were treated with atenolol 50 mg/day. If their recumbent diastolic blood pressure was ≥95 mmHg after 4 weeks, they received either 5, 10, or 20 mg of lisinopril, or placebo, in addition to the atenolol, for an 8-week period. Whereas placebo and 5 mg of lisinopril had no statistical significant effect at trough, the 10- and 20-mg dose of lisinopril reduced recumbent diastolic blood pressure by 3.2 and 3.3 mmHg more than placebo ($p = .01$). The authors pointed out that the combination was of special benefit in younger patients (i.e., less than 50 years), since the decrease in blood pressure observed in this age group was much more pronounced than the reported averages. The combination was well tolerated and although the effects were only modest, the authors recommend consideration of the combination in specific patients. It is important to remember that mean data from groups underestimate the individual effect in responders. In clinical therapy, in contrast to studies, we treat individuals who, when not responding to a drug or drug combination, will be switched to another treatment regimen, whereas those who respond will receive continued treatment. In clinical studies the data of nonresponders dilute the effect of the responders. Conversely, those individual patients who responded had a much stronger response than that indicated by the mean data. It is therefore not justified to conclude from the results of this study that it "failed to confirm additional benefit from such combinations" (37, p.89).

The results must also be seen in the context of intervention studies using major clinical end points. In the meta-analysis by Collins and associates an overall reduction of diastolic blood pressure of about 6 mmHg was associated with a highly significant reduction in stroke (42%) and coronary heart disease (14%) morbidity (38).

STUDIES ON SURROGATE END POINTS

Franz and colleagues (39) have published a study designed to evaluate the long-term effects of a combination between an ACE inhibitor (enalapril 10 mg/day) and a β-blocker (atenolol 50 mg/day) once daily for 39 months. This therapy lowered blood pressure at rest from 161/108 to 130/86 mmHg ($p < .001$) and blood pressure under isotonic (meaning *dynamic*) exercise from 192/112 to 167/95 mmHg ($p < .001$). After 6 months the indices of LVH, especially the left ventricular mass index, were decreased (-16%, $p < .001$) as demonstrated by echocardiography. After 39 months of therapy, reductions amounted to 40%. The authors concluded that a long-term treatment with a combination of atenolol and enalapril produced a pronounced decrease of blood pressure and also a marked reduction of the left ventricular mass. The left ventricular pump function was well preserved at rest and under exercise. The interpretation of the data from that study needs some caution: Since no control groups (e.g., β-blockers or ACE inhibitors alone) had been included, the included benefit of the combination cannot be compared, without reservation, with that obtained in other studies using monotherapies. Nevertheless, the data argue for a long-term efficacy of a β-blocker–ACE inhibitor combination, and of additional hemodynamic and cardioprotective beneficial effects of such a combination.

SUMMARY

The clinical value of a combination of β-blockers and ACE inhibitors in the treatment of hypertension is still controversial, though the majority of published papers reports a somewhat less-than-additive effect of this regimen. The additive antihypertensive effect, as is obvious from the mean data of studies, will somewhat underestimate the effect that may be found in an individual titration experiment in responders. In spite of a similar mechanism of action resulting in a decrease of angiotensin II, there are possible humoral and hemodynamic mechanisms that explain an additivity: The main mechanism may be that the enzymatic activity of chymase is not inhibited by ACE inhibitors and, in the presence of increased angiotensin I concentrations, continued angiotensin II formation will occur. Additional β-blockade reduces the amount of substrate available for this bypass formation of angiotensin II. Conversely, the ACE inhibitor will reduce the vasoconstriction brought about by a β-blocker.

Younger patients with a high renin status and/or high sympathoadrenergic tone and those with exertional hypertension may especially benefit from this combination. In patients after acute myocardial infarction (ACI) it seems conceivable, though not proven, that the combination of β-blockers and ACE inhibitors could not only reduce the risk of subsequent arrhythmias, but also reduce progressive ventricular dilatation and improve exercise tolerance.

Acknowledgment

The author is deeply indebted to his friend Professor Dr. Dieter Palm, University of Frankfurt, for continued stimulation and critical discussion in preparing this manuscript.

REFERENCES

1. Prichard BNC, Gillam PMS. The use of propranolol in the treatment of hypertension. *Br Med J* 1964; 2:725.

2. Palm D. Pharmakologie der antihypertensiva. *Dtsch Apoth Z* 1993; 133:327–336.

3. Brown MJ. To β-block or better block? *Br Med J* 1995; 311:701–702.

4. Belz GG, Breithaupt K, de Mey C. Cholinergic system, heart rate and blood pressure [letter]. *Blood Press* 1992; 1:260.

5. Palm D, Grobecker H. Quantitative parameter der sympatho-nervalen und sympatho-adrenalen aktivatät beim Menschen. Einfluss von β-blockern. *Arzneim Forsch/Drug Res* 1977; 27:708–713.

6. Man in't Veld AJ, Schalekamp ADH. Effects of 10 different beta-Adrenoceptor antagonists on hemodynamics, plasma renin activity, and plasma norepinephrine in hypertension: the key role of vascular resistance changes in relation to partial agonist activity. *J Cardiovasc Pharmacol* 1983; 5:S30–S45.

7. Cruickshank JM, Prichard BNC. *Beta-blockers in clinical practice.* 2nd ed. Edinburgh: Churchill Livingstone, 1994: 106–110, 355–377.

8. Belz GG, Essig A, Wellstein A. Hemodynamic responses to angiotensin-I in normal volunteers and the antagonism by the angiotensin converting enzyme inhibitor cilazapril. *J Cardiovasc Pharmacol* 1987; 9:219–224.

9. Dzau VJ. Circulating versus local renin-angiotensin system in cardiovascular homoeostasis. *Circulation* 1988; 77(Suppl 1):1–4.

10. Peach MJ. Renin-angiotensin system: biochemistry and mechanism of action. *Physiol Rev* 1977; 57:313–337.

11. Williams GM. Converting-enzyme inhibitors in the treatment of hypertension. *N Engl J Med* 1988; 319:1517–1525.

12. Stella A, Macchi A, Genovesi S, et al. Angiotensin converting enzyme inhibition and renin release from the kidney. *J Hypertens* 1989; 7(Suppl 7):S21–S26.

13. Burnier M, Waeber B, Brunner HR. The advantages of angiotensin II antagonism. *J Hypertens* 1994; 12(Suppl 2):S7–S15.

14. Urata H, Strobel F, Ganten D. Widespread tissue distribution of human chymases. *J Hypertens* 1994; 12:S17–S22.

15. Nussberger J, Waeber B, Brunner H. Clinical pharmacology of ACE inhibition. *Cardiology* 1989; 76(Suppl 2):11–22.

16. Stern HC, Matthews JH, Belz GG. Influence of dihydralazine induced afterload reduction on systolic time intervals and echocardiography in healthy subjects. *Br Heart J* 1984; 52:435–439.

17. Stern HC, Matthews JH, Belz GG. Intrinsic and reflex actions of verapamil and nifedipine: assessment in normal subjects by noninvasive techniques and autonomic blockade. *Eur J Clin Pharmacol* 1986; 29:541–547.

18. Hansson L. Beta-blockers with ACE inhibitors—a logical combination? *J Hum Hypertens* 1989; 3:97–100.

19. Staessen J, Fagard R, Lijnen P, et al. The hypotensive effect of propranolol in captopril-treated patients does not involve the plasma renin-angiotensin-aldosterone system. *Clin Sci* 1981; 61:441s–444s.

20. Pickering TG, Case DB, Sullivan PA, Laragh JH. Comparison of antihypertensive and hormonal effects of captopril and propranolol at rest and during exercise. *Am J Cardiol* 1982: 49:1566–1568.

21. MacGregor GA, Markandu ND, Smith SJ, Sagnella GA. Captopril: contrasting effects of adding hydrochlorothiazide, propranolol, or nifedipine. *J Cardiovasc Pharmacol* 1985; 7:S82–S87.

22. Sullivan PA, Daly B, O'Connor R. Enalapril versus combined enalapril and nadolol treatment: effects on blood pressure, heart rate, humoral variables, and plasma potassium at rest and during exercise in hypertensive patients. *Cardiovasc Drugs Ther* 1992; 6:261–265.

23. Belz GG, Essig J, Kleinbloesem CH, et al. Interactions between cilazapril and propranolol in man: plasma drug concentrations, hormone and enzyme responses, haemodynamics, agonist dose-effect curves and baroreceptor reflex. *Br J Clin Pharmacol* 1988; 26:547–556.

24. Belz GG, Essig J, Erb K, et al. Pharmacokinetic and pharmaco-dynamic interactions between the ACE inhibitor cilazapril and β–receptor antagonist propranolol in healthy subjects and in hypertensive patients. *Br J Clin Pharmacol* 1989; 27:S317–S322.

25. Belz GG, Breithaupt K, Erb K, et al. Influence of the ACE inhibitor cilazapril, the β–blocker propranolol and their combination on haemodynamics in hypertension. *J Hypertens* 1989; 7:817–824.

26. Erb KA, Breithaupt K, Kleinbloesem CH, et al. Does the combination of cilazapril and propranolol lower blood pressure at rest and during exercise more pronouncedly than either of the two components given alone? *J Clin Physiol Biochem* 1990; 8(Suppl 2):35–45.

27. van Griensven JMT, Seibert-Grafe M, Schoemaker HC, et al. The pharmacokinetic and pharmacodynamic interactions of ramipril with propranolol. *Eur J Clin Pharmacol* 1993; 45:255–260.

28. Breithaupt K, Belz GG, Spielmanns DG, et al. Antihypertensive treatment with cilazapril resting and exercise blood pressure, hormones and enzymes. *Arzneim Forsch Drug Res* 1990; 40:136–141.

29. Franz IW, Behr U, Ketelhut R. Resting and exercise blood pressure with atenolol, enalapril and a low-dose combination. *J Hypertens* 1987; 5(Suppl 3):S37–S41.

30. Wing LM, Chalmers JP, West MJ, et al. Enalapril and atenolol in essential hypertension: attenuation of hypotensive effect in combination. *Clin Exp Hypertens* 1988; 10:119–133.

31. Soininen K, Gerlin-Piira L, Suihkonen J, et al. A study of the effects of lisinopril when used in addition to atenolol. *J Hum Hypertens* 1992; 6:321–324.

32. Ferguson RK, Vlasses PH, Koffer H, et al. Effect of captopril and propranolol, alone and in combination, on the response to isometric and dynamic exercise in normotensive and hypertensive men. *Pharmacotherapy* 1983; 3:125–130.

33. Lüders S, Schrader J, Scheler F. Kombinationstherapie von β-blockern und ACE-hemmern bei essentieller hypertonie. *Nieren-und Hockdruckkrankheiten* 1992; 21:677–679.

34. Huttunen M, Lampainen E, Lilja M, et al. Which anti-hypertensive to add to a beta-blocker: ACE inhibitor or diuretic? *J Hum Hypertens* 1992; 6:121–125.

35. Bursztyn M, Gavras I, Gourley L, et al. Effect of combination therapy with atenolol and the angiotensin-converting enzyme inhibitor benazepril. *Clin Ther* 1994; 16:429–436.

36. Swedish Lisinopril Study Group. Lisinopril combined with atenolol in the treatment of hypertension. *J Cardiovasc Pharmacol* 1991; 18:457–461.

37. MacConnachie AM, Maclean D. Low dose combination. Antihypertensive therapy: additional efficacy without additional adverse effects? *Drug Safety* 1995; 12:85–90.

38. Collins R, Peto R, MacMahon S, et al. Blood pressure, stroke, and coronary heart disease. *Lancet* 1990; 335:827–838.

39. Ketelhut R, Franz IW, Behr U, et al. Preserved ventricular pump function after a marked reduction of left ventricular mass. *J Am Coll Cardiol* 1992; 20:864–868.

CHAPTER 9

Calcium Antagonists and ACE Inhibitors

*Thomas F. Lüscher, René R. Wenzel,
Pierre Moreau, and Hiroyuki Takase*

Hypertension, although not a disease on its own, is a risk factor for coronary artery disease, stroke, heart failure, and complications in other target organs such as the kidney and the eye (1–4). Many classes of drugs with distinct antihypertensive mechanisms are now available and are generally as equally effective as monotherapy in lowering blood pressure in a significant number of mild to moderate hypertensive patients. Calcium antagonists and ACE inhibitors have been shown to have very good antihypertensive efficacy combined with a low incidence of metabolic side effects (5–8). The combination of these two classes may aim at better controlling the blood pressure in patients resistant to monotherapy or at reducing even further the side effects of the individual compounds, and therefore further improving the quality of life of hypertensive patients (6).

In addition to their antihypertensive efficacy, calcium antagonists and ACE inhibitors have also shown promising and important effects on the vascular function and structures. The antihypertensive and structural effects of these drugs may be directed toward the vascular smooth muscle cells, but may also involve the endothelial cells. Indeed, endothelial cells may play a crucial role in these processes due to their strategic anatomic position between the circulating blood and vascular smooth muscle, and also because of their capacity to release numerous factors regulating the function of vascular smooth muscle cells as well as platelets (9) (Figure 9-1). Among these factors nitric oxide and prostacyclin are particularly important because of their antiplatelet activity and vasodilator properties (10, 11). Furthermore, nitric oxide also has been involved as an antiproliferative principle (12). Endothelin on the other hand is an endothelium-derived vasoconstrictor peptide with proliferative properties (13, 14). This chapter discusses the effects of calcium antagonists and ACE inhibitors, alone or in combination, on endothelium and vascular smooth muscle function with particular emphasis on the effects of nitric oxide, endothelin-1, and angiotensin II.

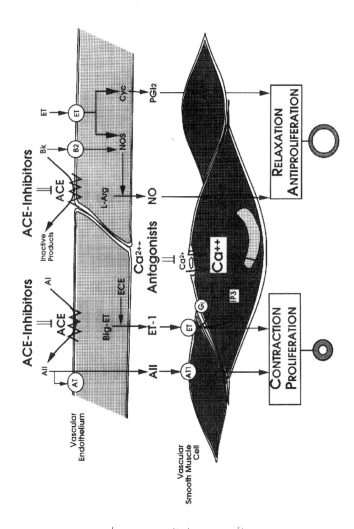

Figure 9-1. Local vascular effects of ACE inhibitors and calcium antagonists. While ACE inhibitors inactivate the formation of angiotensin I (AI) into angiotensin II (AII) as well as the inactivation of bradykinin (Bk) on endothelial cells, Ca²⁺ antagonists primarily interefere with CA²⁺ influx at the level of vascular smooth muscle. AT = angiotensin receptor; cAMP = cyclic 3´, 5´-adenasine monophosphate; cGMP = cyclic 3´, 5´-guanasine monophosphate; CYC = cyclooxygenase; ECE = endothelin-converting enzyme; ET = endothelin; G_i = G_i protein; L-arg = arginine; NO = nitric oxide; NOS = nitric oxide synthase; and PGI₂ = prostacyclin.

CALCIUM ANTAGONISTS

The calcium antagonists have been classified in three main families according to their chemical structure: phenylalkylamines (i.e., verapamil-like), dihydropyridines (i.e., nifedipine-like), and benzothiazepines (i.e., diltiazem-like). All substances interfere with different parts of the voltage-operated, L-type calcium channels, thereby decreasing influx of extracellular calcium into cells, in particular vascular smooth muscle cells. Increases in intracellular calcium is a very basic biological signaling mechanism involving numerous intracellular processes. In the context of hypertension and coronary artery disease, increases in intracellular calcium are particularly important in platelets (leading to platelet activation [15]), in vascular smooth muscle cells (leading to vasoconstriction and proliferation [16]), as well as in endothelial cells (leading to the release of vasoactive substances [17, 18]).

Calcium Antagonists and Endothelium-Dependent Relaxation

The formation of nitric oxide (NO) from its precursor L-arginine occurs via NO-synthases, which can be expressed constitutively (cNOS, for example, in endothelial cells) or which can be induced (iNOS, can be expressed in vascular smooth muscle cells [19–21]). Important stimuli for the synthesis of NO are shear stress, platelet-derived products, coagulation factors, and hormones (22). The formation of NO by cNOS in endothelial cells requires increases in intracellular calcium (19, 20) (see Figure 9-1), which can be mimicked by the calcium ionophore A23187, a very potent activator of NO release (10). In most circumstances calcium antagonists do not affect NO release (23), as endothelial cells do not appear to have voltage-operated calcium channels. However, there may be some effect in perfused arteries (24).

Despite this apparent lack of effect of calcium antagonists on NO release in acute conditions, chronic therapy with calcium antagonists improves endothelium-dependent relaxation to acetylcholine in models of hypertension (25–27). Similarly, in hypercholesterolemic rabbits, the calcium antagonist isradipine improves this response, although it does not restore it completely (28). It is possible that this beneficial response is mediated by more alternative pathways than the L-arginine-NO axis, since verapamil has been shown to enhance endothelium-dependent relaxation in a model of hypertension induced by the chronic blockade of NO synthesis with N^{ω}-nitro-L-arginine methyl ester (L-NAME, an analog of L-arginine) (26, 27) (Figure 9-2). Therefore, despite the deficiency of NO, chronic therapy with verapamil may stimulate a relaxing pathway that is normally overshadowed by the very efficient NO pathway. Although proofs are still lacking, an endothelium-derived hyperpolarizing factor may be involved in this response.

In addition, calcium antagonists may facilitate the effects of NO at the level of vascular smooth muscle cells in certain conditions (23). Indeed, relaxation to the endothe-

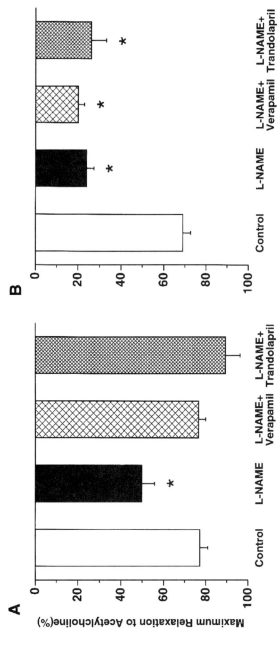

Figure 9-2. Effect of a calcium antagonist and of an ACE inhibitor on endothelium-dependent relaxation of mesenteric resistance arteries from L-NAME-treated rats. (A) Both antihypertensives improved the endothelial function in this model of nitric oxide synthase blockade when they were administered chronically for 6 weeks. (B) In contrast, the same drugs were ineffective when applied acutely for 30 minutes in the organ bath (modified from Takase and associates [27]). *p < .05, as compared to control animals.

lium-independent vasodilator (a NO donor) sodium nitro-
prusside is sometimes augmented (23).

Calcium Antagonists and Endothelin

The production of endothelin in endothelial cells is also associated with an increased intracellular calcium (18) (see
Figure 9-1). Indeed, the calcium ionophore A23187 is a very
potent stimulator of endothelin production (18). However,
calcium antagonists do not modulate endothelin production
in vitro or in vivo, as exemplified by the lack of effect of
nifedipine on the increased plasma endothelin levels induced by high altitude in healthy mountaineers (29).

Although originally considered an endogenous activator of voltage-operated calcium channels (14), more recent
data have demonstrated that endothelin interacts with specific receptors on vascular smooth muscle cells mediating
vasoconstriction and proliferation (30) through ET_A- and ET_B-
receptors (31–34), as well as on endothelial cells to stimulate
the formation of NO and prostacylin through ET_B-receptors
(32, 33, 35) (see Figure 9-1). In certain blood vessels such as
the porcine coronary artery, the endothelin receptors on vascular smooth muscle cells are linked to voltage-operated calcium channels via G_i-proteins (36). This may explain why
calcium antagonists do reduce endothelin-induced vasoconstriction in this blood vessel. As calcium antagonists are also
effective in the human coronary artery (37), the same mechanism may also be operative in humans. However, in the human internal mammary artery the contractile effects of
endothelin appear to be mediated via a cascade activation of
phospholipase C, diacylglycerol, and ultimately inositol
triphosphate that, in turn, releases calcium from the sarco-
plasmic reticulum and therefore increases cytosolic calcium
(38–40). This may explain why calcium antagonists of all
classes are unable to prevent endothelin-induced contractions in this artery (38). On the other hand, in veins, calcium
antagonists are able to reverse, at least in part, endothelin-
induced contractions (38, 41). This is most likely related to
the fact that endothelin lowers the membrane potential of
venous vascular smooth muscle cells (41) and thereby opens
voltage-operated calcium channels. Hence, once contractions
have developed, calcium antagonists do exert an inhibitory
effect due to this phenomenon.

Several studies have suggested that small vessels are
more dependent than larger vessels on the influx of extracellular calcium for contraction (16, 42). Indeed, in human forearm circulation, intra-arterial application of verapamil or
nifedipine prevents contractions to endothelin infused by
the same route (43) (Figure 9-3), and even unmasks the vasodilator effects of endothelin. However, particularly with
higher concentrations of endothelin-1, oral administration
of verapamil does not appear to be effective enough to reduce endothelin-induced contractions (unpublished observation, Kiowski W, Linder L, and Lüscher TF, 1996). Hence,
higher local concentration of the drugs may be required to
inhibit fully vasoconstriction induced by this potent biological peptide. It is therefore uncertain at this stage whether the

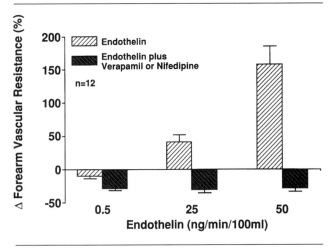

Figure 9-3. Effects of endothelin-1 in the human forearm circulation in the presence and absence of the Ca2+ antagonists verapamil or nifedipine. The results of two series of experiments with the two Ca²⁺ antagonists have been pooled as similar results have been obtained. The change in forearm blood vascular resistance is given. Both nifedipine and verapamil fully prevented the decrease in forearm vascular resistance occurring with higher concentrations of endothelin and, en masse, the vasodilator effects of the peptide. (From Kiowski and coworkers [43], with permission of the American Heart Associaton.)

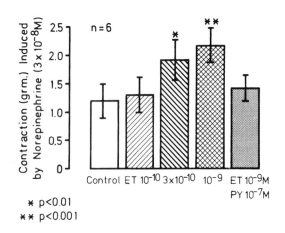

Figure 9-4. Effects of threshold concentrations of endothelin-1 (10^{-10} $-10^{-9}M$) on the contractions to norepinephrine ($3 \times 10^{-8} M$) in human mammary artery rings. The contractions to norepinephrine are significantly augmented in the presence of threshold concentrations of endothelin-1. The dihydropyridine calcium antagonist darodipine (PY) prevents this effect. (From Yang and colleagues [42] with permission of the American Heart Association.)

usual clinical oral dosage of verapamil or nifedipine is sufficient to inhibit endogenous endothelin-mediated contractions. Such studies would be necessary to determine the potential usefulness of calcium antagonists in clinical disease states associated with increased endothelin production.

In addition to its direct vasoconstriction, endothelin potentiates contraction to other agonists, such as serotonin and norepinephrine, even at subthreshold concentrations for direct contraction (42). This has been shown in human internal mammary and coronary arteries. The mechanism underlying this amplifying effect seems to be an increased sensitivity of the vascular smooth muscle cell to calcium and it can be prevented by a calcium antagonist of the dihydropyridine type (42) (Figure 9-4).

ACE INHIBITORS

The renin-angiotensin system is an important regulator of the cardiovascular system (44, 45), and evidence has accumulated to suggest that it is both a circulating and a local vascular system. The endothelial cells express the ACE (46), which transforms angiotensin I into angiotensin II (9) (see Figure 9-1). In addition, other parts of the renin-angiotensin system are also expressed in endothelial cells, although the physiological importance of these findings has not been yet established. Similarly, vascular smooth muscle cells do express components of the renin-angiotensin system (45). Due to the interaction of the renin-angiotensin system with local autacoids, ACE inhibitors can also modulate the action of other substances involved in endothelium-dependent regulation of vascular tone, such as bradykinin and substance P (9) (see Figure 9-1).

ACE Inhibitors and Endothelium-Derived Relaxing Factor

Under most circumstances, acute pretreatment of isolated blood vessels with an ACE inhibitor does not affect endothelium-dependent relaxation to acetylcholine (47), although it may do so during chronic therapy (48). However, the response to bradykinin, which also acts primarily by stimulating the production of NO, is profoundly affected by ACE inhibitors (49–54). Indeed, pretreatment of human saphenous veins or coronary arteries with enalapril markedly increases the sensitivity to bradykinin, indicating that the endothelial ACE continually inactivates part of the bradykinin added to the blood vessel (52, 55). Similarly, in the perfused porcine eye, ACE inhibitors markedly enhance the increase in ophthalmic flow induced by bradykinin (56) (Figure 9-5). In contrast, in the human internal mammary artery, ACE activity does not seem to be as marked (52). Therefore there may be regional vascular heterogeneity in ACE activity or expression. It cannot be excluded, however, that the capacity to inhibit the vascular renin-angiotensin system differs between ACE inhibitors. Indeed, in human forearm circulation, intra-arterial infusion of enalapril or captopril does not increase local blood flow, while the highly tissue-selective ACE inhibitor quinaprilat increases forearm blood flow, most likely by activating the L-arginine pathway secondary to the prevention of bradykinin breakdown (57).

In experimental models of hypertension, chronic therapy with ACE inhibitors augments endothelium-depen-

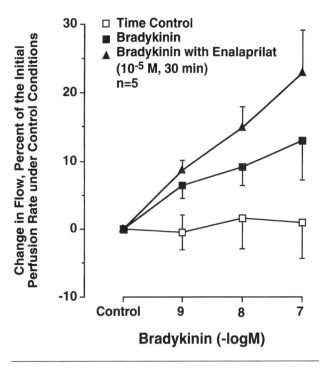

Figure 9-5. *Effect of enalaprilat on endothelium-dependent vasodilation in the perfused porcine eye. Bradykinin caused concentration-dependent increases in ophthalmic flow that were enhanced in the presence of the ACE inhibitor. (From Meyer and colleagues (56), with permission.)*

dent relaxation not only to bradykinin, but also to other agonists such as acetylcholine (see Figure 9-2). This effect can be demonstrated in large conduit arteries (26) as well as in mesenteric resistance arteries (27, 58). As this endothelial protective effect can be obtained with different ACE inhibitors such as benazapril and trandolapril (27, 58, 59), it appears to be a common property of this class. It is possible that this improvement of endothelium-dependent relaxations during chronic therapy is secondary to the protection of bradykinin breakdown. In that context, it is of particular interest that endothelial cells can produce and release bradykinin locally, particularly in response to flow (most likely due to the shear forces exerted by the circulating blood [17, 54, 60]). As with calcium antagonists, chronic administration of an ACE inhibitor also improves the endothelial function of rats treated with L-NAME, an inhibitor of NO synthase (26, 27) (see Figure 9-2). It is therefore possible that an alternative pathway to L-arginine-NO may be stimulated with chronic ACE inhibitor therapy. As previously discussed with calcium antagonists, the endothelial hyperpolarizing factor (EDHF) may be involved and, interestingly, bradykinin also stimulates this pathway (61). Whatever the mediator, the process seems to require some time to develop, since a 30-minute preincubation of L-NAME-treated vessels with an ACE inhibitor or with a calcium antagonist does not improve endothelium-dependent relaxation as compared to L-NAME alone (27) (see Figure 9-2).

In hypertensive subjects, two studies have reported the effects of captopril, enalapril (62), and cilazapril (personal communication with Kiowski and Linder, 1992) on endothelium-dependent vasodilatation to acetylcholine in forearm circulation. In contrast to the experimental data in the rat, ACE inhibitors were unable to normalize or even to improve the impaired endothelium-dependent vasodilatation of these patients. This lack of effect may be related to the duration of therapy (less than 6 months), to the time when therapy was started, and/or to the ineffectiveness of this approach in humans. Hence, studies with more prolonged and early treatment with ACE inhibitors are required to reach a final conclusion on these effects of the drugs. In addition, the elucidation of the mechanism of endothelial improvement in the rat may be important to determine how this pathway could be stimulated in humans, if at all present.

ACE Inhibitors and Endothelin-1

Angiotensin II has been shown to increase the expression of endothelin messenger ribonucleic acid (mRNA) in endothelial cells in culture (9, 14, 47). In addition, angiotensin II appears to exert similar effects in endothelial cells obtained from the rat mesenteric microcirculation (47). Expression of endothelin in response to angiotensin II may contribute to the vasoconstrictor effects of angiotensin. Indeed, endothelin antagonists have been shown to blunt angiotensin II-induced contractions, especially in conduit arteries of smaller caliber (63) and in resistance vessels (64). In addition, endothelin may also mediate the amplification of norepinephrine contractions observed after angiotensin II pretreatment (64). Indeed, this effect of angiotensin II is endothelium dependent and can be inhibited by endothelin antibodies and inhibitors of the endothelin-converting enzymes such as phosophoramidon. Hence, it appears that angiotensin II stimulates the local vascular production of endothelin and thereby enhances responses to noradrenaline and possibly to other endogenous vasoconstrictors. Although this hypothesis deserves direct support, it is reasonable to think that ACE inhibitors, by preventing the formation of angiotensin II, could also decrease the influence of endothelin on vascular function.

COMBINATION OF CALCIUM ANTAGONISTS AND ACE INHIBITORS

Although blood pressure lowering is possible with almost all antihypertensive drugs available on the market, it may be advantageous to use combination therapy, provided the two drugs selected act on different regulatory processes of the circulation. This may provide better hemodynamic as well as vascular protective effects. A further advantage of combination therapy would be a reduction in the dosage and side effects of each individual drug. Both ACE inhibitors and calcium antagonists have been shown to be effective in lowering blood pressure in patients with essential hypertension

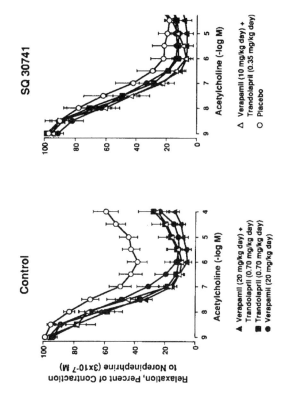

Figure 9-6. Effects of chronic therapy with verapamil or trandolapril alone or in combination on endothelium-dependent relaxations in the aorta of stroke-prone, spontaneously hypertensive rats (SHR-SP). Responses were impaired in untreated SHR-SP as compared to normotensive rats (not shown) and enhanced to a similar degree by chronic therapy with a high dose of verapamil or trandolapril alone or by combination therapy of the two drugs. Most interestingly the low-dose combination therapy was as effective as the high-dose combination therapy. SQ30741 = thromboxane receptor antagonist. (From Novosel and colleagues [59] with permisson.)

(44). Conceptually, a combination of the two drugs could be advantageous, as they are indeed interfering with different regulatory mechanisms. Calcium antagonists are very potent vasodilators, as shown by the 8- to10-fold increase in forearm blood flow when these compounds are infused locally (43). In contrast, ACE inhibitors do not cause marked vasodilatation with a few exceptions (57; see earlier discussion), but interfere with the renin-angiotensin system, an important regulatory pathway for vascular function and structure. Furthermore, calcium antagonists stimulate the sympathetic nervous system (65), while ACE inhibitors reduce sympathetic activity (66). The combination may prove to be interesting in that respect.

Of particular interest in the context of endothelial dysfunction in hypertension is the finding that the combination of low-dose ACE inhibitors and calcium antagonists seems to be as effective as high-dose monotherapy to improve endothelium-dependent relaxation in hypertensive animals (48) (Figure 9-6). The proper combination of these two classes of antihypertensive drugs, rather than monotherapy, may therefore be required to normalize the endothelial dysfunction in hypertensive patients who seem to be resistant to ACE inhibitors used alone. The effect of these two classes of drugs on the endothelin axis also deserves special attention. Indeed, very high local concentrations of calcium antagonists seem to be required to blunt the potent vasoconstriction induced by the peptide, especially at high local concentrations. The partial inhibition of endothelin synthesis by ACE inhibitors could reduce local endothelin concentrations, thus enhancing the effect of calcium antagonists.

Impaired renal function is an important complication of hypertension, diabetes, and atherosclerotic vascular disease. Particularly in diabetes, but also in hypertension, an increased intraglomerular pressure has accounted for damage to the kidney (67). Albumin excretion has been used as a surrogate marker to determine changes in early renal damage during therapy with calcium antagonists or ACE inhibitors (68, 69). ACE inhibitors are particularly interesting in this context as they primarily lower efferent renal resistance and hence most effectively reduce intraglomerular pressure. However, calcium antagonists also lower intraglomerular pressure by reducing perfusion pressure and both afferent and efferent renal resistance. Clinical trials have shown that albumin excretion is reduced with chronic therapy with an ACE inhibitor as well as with a calcium antagonist such as verapamil. Combination therapy seems to have an additive effect (70). Therefore, the combination of a calcium antagonist and an ACE inhibitor is promising in patients with impaired renal function, particularly when other factors such as hypertension are associated.

CONCLUSION

Vascular protection aims at reducing the incidence of cardiovascular complications of hypertension beyond blood pressure control alone. Calcium antagonists and ACE inhibitors are not only potent antihypertensive drugs, but they have been shown to exert vascular protective effects, both experimentally and in patients. The combination of the two classes appears promising from the global hemodynamic point of view as well as from the local vascular and endothelial perspective. These concepts, based on currently available observations with either class of drugs studied alone, deserve testing both in experimental models and in humans. Combination therapy should not only enhance antihypertensive efficacy and vascular protection, but should also allow reduction of the doses of each individual drug and thereby the incidence of side effects. Indeed, quality of life is an important issue, especially in hypertensive subjects who are generally asymptomatic.

Acknowledgment

Research was supported by grants of the Swiss National Research Foundation (No. 32-32562.91), the Mobiliar Insurance Foundation, Patria Insurances, as well as by a grant-in-aid of Knoll Pharmaceuticals AG, Ludwigshafen, Germany.

René R. Wenzel is the recipient of a stipend of the German Research Association (Deutsche Forschungsgemeinschaft (DFG), We 17 72/1-1). Pierre Moreau receives a fellowship from the Medical Research Council of Canada.

REFERENCES

1. Kannel WB, Gordon T, Schwartz MJ. Systolic versus diastolic blood pressure and risk of coronary heart disease. The Framingham study. *Am J Cardiol* 1971; 27:335–346.

2. Kannel WB, Castelli WP, McNamara PM, et al. Role of blood pressure in the development of congestive heart failure. The Framingham study. *N Engl J Med* 1972; 287:781–787,

3. Garcia-Cosmes P, Mortezo A, Lopez-Novoa JM, Macias-Nunez JF. Is renal protection with calcium antagonists possible? *Drugs* 1992; 44:99–102.

4. Klag MJ, Whelton PK, Randall BL, et al. Blood pressure and end-stage renal disease in men. *N Engl J Med* 1996; 334:13–18.

5. Lüscher TF, Waeber B. Calcium antagonists as first-line therapy in hypertension: results of the Swiss Isradipine Study. Swiss Hypertension Society. *J Cardiovasc Pharmacol* 1991; 18 (Suppl 3):S1–S3.

6. Lüscher TF, Waeber B. Efficacy and safety of various combination therapies based on a calcium antagonist in essential hypertension: results of a placebo-controlled randomized trial. *J Cardiovasc Pharmacol* 1993; 21:305–309.

7. Weinberger MH. Calcium antagonists for the treatment of systemic hypertension. *Am J Cardiol* 1992; 69:13E–16E.

8. Fröhlich ED. Obesity hypertension. Converting enzyme inhibitors and calcium antagonists. *Hypertension* 1992; 19:119–123.

9. Ross R. The pathogenesis of atherosclerosis: a perspective for the 1990s. *Nature* 1993; 362:801–809.

10. Furchgott RF, Zawadzki JV. The obligatory role of endothelial cells in the relaxation of arterial smooth muscle by acetylcholine. *Nature* 1980; 288:373–376.

11. Radomski MW, Palmer RM, Moncada S. The anti-aggregating properties of vascular endothelium: interactions between prostacyclin and nitric oxide. *Br J Pharmacol* 1987; 92:639–646.

12. Garg UC, Hassid A. Nitric oxide-generating vasodilators and 8-bromo-cyclic guanosine monophosphate inhibit mitogenesis and proliferation of cultured rat vascular smooth muscle cells. *J Clin Invest* 1989; 83:1774–1777.

13. Yanagisawa M, Inoue A, Ishikawa T, et al. Primary structure, synthesis, and biological activity of rat endothelin, an endothelium-derived vasoconstrictor peptide. *Proc Natl Acad Sci USA* 1988; 85:6964–6967.

14. Yanagisawa M, Kurihara H, Kimura S, et al. A novel potent vasoconstrictor peptide produced by vascular endothelial cells. *Nature* 1988; 332:411–415.

15. Erne P, Bolli P, Burgisser E, Buhler FR. Correlation of platelet calcium with blood pressure. Effect of antihypertensive therapy. *N Engl J Med* 1984; 310:1084–1088.

16. Cauvin C, Tejerina M, Hwang O, et al. The effects of Ca2+-antagonists on isolated rat and rabbit mesenteric resistance vessels. What determines the sensitivity of agonist-activated vessels to Ca2+-antagonists? *Ann N Y Acad Sci* 1988; S22:338–350.

17. Busse R, Lamontagne D. Endothelium-derived bradykinin is responsible for the increase in calcium produced by angiotensin-converting enzyme inhibitors in human endothelial cells. *Naunyn Schmiedebergs Arch Pharmacol* 1991; 344:126–129.

18. Boulanger C, Lüscher TF. Release of endothelin from the porcine aorta. Inhibition by endothelium-derived nitric oxide. *J Clin Invest* 1990; 85:587–590.

19. Palmer RM, Ashton DS, Moncada S. Vascular endothelial cells synthesize nitric oxide from L-arginine. *Nature* 1988; 333:664–666.

20. Bredt DS, Hwang PM, Glatt CE, et al. Cloned and expressed nitric oxide synthase structurally resembles cytochrome P-450 reductase. *Nature* 1991; 351:714–718.

21. Radomski MW, Palmer RM, Moncada S. Glucocorticoids inhibit the expression of an inducible, but not the constitutive, nitric oxide synthase in vascular endothelial cells. *Proc Natl Acad Sci* USA 1990; 87:1043–1047.

22. Lüscher TF. Endothelium-derived nitric oxide: the endogenous nitrovasodilator in the human cardiovascular system. *Eur Heart J* 1991; 12:2–11.

23. Küng CF, Tschudi MR, Noll G, et al. Differential effects of the calcium antagonist mibefradil in epicardial and intramyocardial coronary arteries. *J Cardiovasc Pharmacol* 1995; 26:312–318.

24. Rubanyi GM, Schwartz A, Vanhoutte PM. The calcium agonists Bay K 8644 and (+)202,791 stimulate the release of endothelial relaxing factor from canine femoral arteries. *Eur J Pharmacol* 1985; 117:143–144.

25. Tschudi MR, Criscione L, Novosel D, et al. Antihypertensive therapy augments endothelium-dependent relaxations in coronary arteries of spontaneously hypertensive rats. *Circulation* 1994; 89:2212–2218.

26. Küng CF, Moreau P, Takase H, Lüscher TF. L-NAME hypertension alters endothelial and smooth muscle function in rat aorta. Prevention by trandolapril and verapamil. *Hypertension* 1995; 26:744–751.

27. Takase H, Moreau P, Küng CF, et al. Antihypertensive therapy

prevents endothelial dysfunction in chronic nitric oxide deficiency: effect of verapamil and trandolapril. *Hypertension* 1996:27:25–31.

28. Henry PD, Bentley KI. Suppression of atherogenesis in cholesterol-fed rabbit treated with nifedipine. *J Clin Invest* 1981; 68:1366–1369.

29. Goerre S, Wenk M, Bärtsch P, et al. Endothelin-1 in pulmonary hypertension associated with high altitude. *Circulation* 1994; 90:359–364.

30. Hirata Y, Takagi Y, Fukuda Y, Marumo F. Endothelin is a potent mitogen for rat vascular smooth muscle cells. *Atherosclerosis* 1989; 78:225–228.

31. Arai H, Hori S, Aramori I, et al. Cloning and expression of a cDNA encoding an endothelin receptor [see comments]. *Nature* 1990; 348:730–732.

32. Sakurai T, Yanagisawa M, Takuwa Y, et al. Cloning of a cDNA encoding a non-isopeptide-selective subtype of the endothelin receptor [see comments]. *Nature* 1990; 348:732–735.

33. Vane J. Endothelins come home to roost [news; comment]. *Nature* 1990; 348:973–975.

34. Seo BG, Oemar BS, Siebenmann R, et al. Both ETA and ETB receptors mediate contraction to endothelin-1 in human blood vessels. *Circulation* 1994; 89:1203–1208.

35. Dohi Y, Lüscher TF. Endothelin in hypertensive resistance arteries. Intraluminal and extraluminal dysfunction. *Hypertension* 1991; 18:543–549.

36. Goto K, Kasuya Y, Matsuki N, et al. Endothelin activates the dihydropyridine-sensitive, voltage-dependent Ca(2+) channel in vascular smooth muscle. *Proc Natl Acad Sci USA* 1989; 86:3915–3918.

37. Godfraind T, Mennig D, Morel N, Wibo M. Effect of endothelin-1 on calcium channel gating by agonists in vascular smooth muscle. *J Cardiovasc Pharmacol* 1989; 13:S112–S117.

38. Yang Z, Bauer E, Von Segesser L, et al. Different mobilization of calcium in endothelin-1-induced contractions in human arteries and veins: effects of calcium antagonists. *J Cardiovasc Pharmacol* 1990; 16:654–660.

39. Resink TJ, Scott-Burden T, Bühler FR. Endothelin stimulates phospholipase C in cultured vascular smooth muscle cells. *Biochem Biophys Res Commun* 1988; 157:1360–1368.

40. Wallnöfer A, Weir S, Ruegg U, Cauvin C. The mechanism of action of endothelin-1 as compared with other agonists in vascular smooth muscle. *J Cardiovasc Pharmacol* 1989; 13(Suppl 5):S23–S31.

41. Miller VM, Komori K, Burnett Jr JC, Vanhoutte PM. Differential sensitivity to endothelin in canine arteries and veins. *Am J Physiol* 1989; 257:H11127–H1131.

42. Yang ZH, Richard V, Von Segesser L, et al. Threshold concentrations of endothelin-1 potentiate contractions to norepinephrine and serotonin in human arteries. A new mechanism of vasospasm? *Circulation* 1990; 82:188–95.

43. Kiowski W, Lüscher TF, Linder L, Bühler FR. Endothelin-1-induced vasoconstriction in humans. Reversal by calcium channel blockade but not by nitrovasodilators or endothelium-derived relaxing factor. *Circulation* 1991; 83:469–475.

44. Sealey JE, Laragh HH. The renin angiotensin aldosterone system for normal regulation of blood pressure and sodium and potassium homeostasis. In: Laragh JH, Brenner BM, eds. *Hypertension, pathophysiology, diagnosis and management.* New York: Raven Press, 1990:1287–1317.

45. Dzau VJ. Short- and long-term determinants of cardiovascular function and therapy: contributions of circulating and tissue renin-angiotensin systems. *J Cardiovasc Pharmacol* 1989; 14:S1–S5.

46. Caldwell PR, Seegal BC, Hsu KC, et al. Angiotensin-converting enzyme: vascular endothelial localization. *Science* 1976; 191:1050–1051.

47. Dohi Z, Hahn AWA, Boulanger CM, Lüscher TF. Vascular renin angiotensin system and endothelial function: effect of ACE-inhibitors. In: MacGregor EA, Safar PS, Caldwell D, Hollenberg NK, eds., *Current advance in ACE-inhibition II*. Edinburgh: Churchill Livingstone, 1991: 226–229.

48. Bossaller C, Auch-Schwelk W, Weber F, et al. Endothelium-dependent relaxations are augmented in rats chronically treated with the angiotensin-converting enzyme inhibitor enalapril. *J Cardiovasc Pharmacol* 1992; 20(Suppl 9):S91–S95.

49. Mombouli JV, Nephtali M, Vanhoutte PM. Effects of the converting enzyme inhibitor cilazaprilat on endothelium-dependent responses. *Hypertension* 1991; 18:1122–1129.

50. Feletou M, Germain M, Teisseire B. Converting-enzyme inhibitors potentiate bradykinin-induced relaxation in vitro. *Am J Physiol* 1990; 262:H839–H845.

51. Feletou M, Teisseire B. Converting enzyme inhibition in isolated porcine resistance artery potentiates bradykinin relaxation. *Eur J Pharmacol* 1990; 190:159–166.

52. Yang Z, Arnet U, von Segesser L, et al. Different effects of angiotensin-converting enzyme inhibition in human arteries and veins. *J Cardiovasc Pharmacol* 1993; 22:17–22.

53. Auch-Schwelk W, Bossaller C, Claus M, Graf K, Grafe M, Fleck E. ACE inhibitors are endothelium dependent vasodilators of coronary arteries during submaximal stimulation with bradykinin. *Cardiovasc Res* 1993; 27:312–317.

54. Wiemer G, Scholkens BA, Becker RH, Busse R. Ramiprilat enhances endothelial autacoid formation by inhibiting breakdown of endothelium-derived bradykinin. *Hypertension* 1991; 18:588–563.

55. Auch-Schwelk W, Bossaller C, Claus M, et al. Local potentiation of bradykinin-induced vasodilation by converting-enzyme inhibition in isolated coronary arteries. *J Cardiovasc Pharmacol* 1992; 20:S62–S67.

56. Meyer P, Flammer J, Lüscher TF. Local action of the renin angiotensin system in the porcine ophthalmic circulation: effects of ACE-inhibitors and angiotensin receptor antagonists. *Invest Ophthal Vis Sci* 1995; 36:555–562.

57. Haefeli WE, Linder L, Lüscher TF. Effects of inhibition of tissue angiotensin-converting enzyme with quinaprilat on bradykinin-induced relaxation in the human forearm circulation in vivo. *Hypertension* 1996 (resubmitted).

58. Dohi Y, Criscione L, Pfeiffer M, Lüscher TF. Angiotensin blockade or calcium antagonists improve endothelial dysfunction in hypertension: studies in perfused mesenteric resistance arteries. *J Cardiovasc Pharmacol* 1994; 24:372–379.

59. Novosel D, Lang MG, Noll G, Lüscher TF. Endothelial dysfunction in aorta of the spontaneously hypertensive, stroke-prone rat: effects of therapy with verapamil and trandolapril alone and in combination. *J Cardiovasc Pharmacol* 1994; 24:979–985.

60. Bogle RG, Coade SB, Moncada S, et al. Bradykinin and ATP stimulate L-arginine uptake and nitric oxide release in vascular endothelial cells. *Biochem Biophys Res Commun* 1991; 180:926–932.

61. Feletou M, Vanhoutte PM. Endothelium-dependent hyperpolarization of canine coronary smooth muscle. *Br J Pharmacol* 1988; 93:515–524.

62. Creager MA, Roddy MA, Coleman SM, Dzau VJ. The effect of ACE-inhibition on endolthelium-dependent vasodilation in hypertension. *J Vasc Res* 1992; 29:97–101.

63. Chen L, McNeill JR, Wilson TW, Gopalakrishnan LV. Heterogeneity in vascular smooth muscle responsiveness to angiotensin II: role of endothelin. *Hypertension* 1995; 26:83–88.

64. Dohi Y, Hahn AW, Boulanger CM, et al. Endothelin stimulated by angiotensin II augments contractility of spontaneously hypertensive rat resistance arteries. *Hypertension* 1992; 19:131–137.

65. Wenzel RR, Binggeli C, Lüscher TF, Noll G. Differential activation of cardiac and peripheral sympathetic nervous system by nifedipine: effects of pharmacokinetics and sympathetic stimulation. *Circulation* 1995; (submitted for publication).

66. Noll G, Wenzel RR, De Marchi S, Lüscher TF. Differential effects of nitrate and captopril on muscle sympathetic nerve activity. *Circulation* 1996; (submitted for publication).

67. Hollenberg NK, Raij L. Angiotensin-converting enzyme inhibition and renal protection. An assessment of implications for therapy. *Arch Intern Med* 1993; 153:2426–2435.

68. Bigazzi R, Bianchi S, Baldari D, et al. Microalbuminuria in salt-sensitive patients. A marker for renal and cardiovascular risk factors. *Hypertension* 1994; 23:195–199.

69. Mimran A, Ribstein J, Du Cailar G. Is microalbuminuria a marker of early intrarenal vascular dysfunction in essential hypertension? *Hypertension* 1994; 23:1018–1021.

70. Fioretto P, Frigato F, Velussi M, et al. Effects of angiotensin converting enzyme inhibitors and calcium antagonists on atrial natriuretic peptide release and action and on albumin excretion rate in hypertensive insulin-dependent diabetic patients. *Am J Hypertens* 1992; 5:837–846.

CHAPTER 10

Alpha-Blocker Combinations

Norman M. Kaplan

Before presenting the evidence for the use of alpha-blockers in combination for the treatment of hypertension, a brief review of the current status of alpha-blocker therapy in general seems appropriate. In brief, these drugs—now three in number—despite their many attractive features, are not among the more popular agents being prescribed today. Even though they were recommended by the JNC in the same manner as were ACE inhibitors and calcium antagonists (1), these latter classes are much more popular than alpha-blockers.

THE UNFULFILLED PROMISE

As we noted a few years ago, there are multiple reasons why alpha-blocker therapy of hypertension is "an unfulfilled promise" (2). These include:

- a perception that they have less antihypertensive efficacy and that tolerance to the efficacy often develops
- concern about first-dose syncope and subsequent hypotension
- the late appreciation of their lipid and hormonal benefits long after these drugs were no longer "state of the art"
- the limited number of this class, so that their marketing was overwhelmed by the numerous ACE inhibitors and calcium antagonists

Nonetheless, alpha-blockers do provide some special advantages and their use should increase for these reasons:

1. As shown in the only long-term trial of monotherapy with one of each of the five major classes of drugs, the 4-year TOMH study (3), an alpha-blocker was equally effective as the other drugs and no tolerance developed.
2. The newer agents, doxazosin and terazosin, have a slower onset and longer duration of action so that initial hypotension is very rare and once-a-day dosing is possible.

3. Increasingly strong evidence documents the abililty of alpha-blockers to improve lipid status (4) and insulin sensitivity (5), a combination that is unique among all antihypertensive choices.
4. Alpha-blockers are now recognized as relieving the obstructive symptoms of benign prostatic hypertrophy so well that they are recommended as the first choice of therapy for many patients with prostatism (6).
5. Alpha-blockers are specifically effective in blocking the peripheral vasoconstriction induced by nicotine (7) and allow full cardiovascular responses to exercise (8), particularly in comparison to beta-blockers.

These multiple benefits, some unique to this group of drugs, presages their increased use. When given alone, they are equally effective as other classes of drugs (3), so that perhaps half of hypertensives could be adequately treated with an alpha-blocker alone. However for many, if not most, a combination will be needed.

ALPHA-BLOCKER PLUS DIURETIC

This combination will be the most commonly used, largely because of the widening realization that most hypertensives will need the slight volume contraction that can only be provided by a diuretic to provide the full antihypertensive effect of whatever else is used to treat hypertension. Reactive sodium retention certainly can follow the institution of alpha-blocker therapy (9). Therefore, the addition of a small dose of a diuretic should and does enhance the efficacy of the alpha-blocker while mitigating the adverse metabolic effects of the diuretic (10).

TABLE 10-1. SUPINE AND STANDING SYSTOLIC (S) AND DIASTOLIC (D) BLOOD PRESSURE (BP) AT THE START AND AT THE END OF 12 WEEKS OF TREATMENT WITH DOXAZOSIN/ ATENOLOL (D) (N = 38) AND PLACEBO/ATENOLOL (P) (N = 36)

		Start	End	Mean Change (SD)
Standing SBP (mmHg)	D	161	144	−17 (2.7)*
	P	158	152	−6 (2.9)
Standing DBP (mmHg)	D	107	94	−12 (1.5)*
	P	106	99	−7 (1.7)
Supine SBP (mmHG)	D	162	148	−13 (2.4)
	P	160	151	−9 (3.1)
Supine DBP (mmHg)	D	103	93	−10 (1.3)**
	P	101	95	−6(1.5)

*$p < .05$.
**$p = .05$ between groups.
SD = standard deviation.
(From Searle and colleagues [11], with permission.)

ALPHA-BLOCKER PLUS BETA-BLOCKER

The addition of an alpha-blocker to a beta-blocker lowers the blood pressure significantly. In a double-blind study of 87 patients taking atenolol 100 mg, 44 patients were randomly assigned to doxazosin (mean dose, 11 mg a day), the others to placebo. After 12 weeks, the 38 who remained on the combination had significantly lower blood pressures than did the 36 on beta-blocker plus placebo (Table 10-1). The authors conclude that, "Doxazosin proved to be well tolerated and effective in patients with blood pressure refractory to atenolol aone" (11).

Similar findings were noted when terazosin was added to atenolol (12). In this 8-week study, the alpha-blocker induced beneficial effects on serum lipids compared to the adverse effects seen with beta-blocker plus placebo.

ALPHA-BLOCKER AND ACE INHIBITOR

In a double-blind crossover study, 9 hypertensives were given 4 weeks of either doxazosin (1 to 4 mg) or enalapril (5 to 20 mg) or a combination of the two (1 mg doxazosin and 5 mg enalapril) with 2-week intervals between the three regimens (13). Synergism was found with greater falls in pressure with the combination despite the use of only the median dose of each drug reached at the end of the 2-week dose titration rather than the larger doses during single therapy (Table 10-2).

In two later studies, doxazosin in combination with enalapril provided additive but not synergistic effects (14, 15). The combination was well tolerated.

ALPHA-BLOCKER AND CALCIUM ANTAGONIST

Starting with prazosin (16) and progressing to doxazosin (17) and terazosin (18), alpha-blockers have been found to work well with calcium antagonists, providing additive antihypertensive effects with only occasional orthostatic symptoms. The meticulous studies by both Donnelly and colleagues (17) and Lenz and associates (18) found no significant pharmacokinetic or pharmacodynamic interactions.

TABLE 10-2. CHANGES IN BLOOD PRESSURE AT THE END OF EACH TREATMENT PHASE*

	Doxazosin	Enalapril	Combination
MD (mg)	4	20	1 + 5
S (mmHg)	$7 \pm 7/4 \pm 8$	$14 \pm 14/5 \pm 8$	$23 \pm 12/15 \pm 7$
E (mmHg)	$12 \pm 15/8 \pm 9$	$9 \pm 11/6 \pm 5$	$23 \pm 17/20 \pm 12$

*Mean ± standard deviation.
MD = median dose; S = supine; E = erect.
(From Brown and Dickerson [13], with permission.)

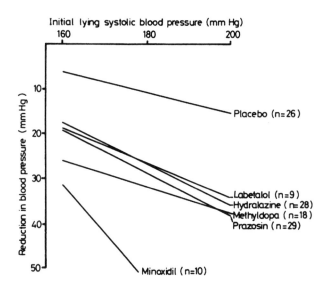

Figure 10-1. Regression lines relating reduction in blood pressure to initial lying systolic pressure for each drug group in randomized trial of placebo and five drugs in patients whose diastolic blood pressure remained >95 on diuretic and β-blocker. N = number of patients in each group who were able to complete the study. (From McAreavey and colleagues [20], with permission.)

ALPHA-BLOCKERS VERSUS OTHER DRUGS

In a VA cooperative study, a representative of all the major classes of drugs was randomly given initially as monotherapy to about 200 each of 1,292 men with initial diastolic blood pressure from 95 to 109 mmHg (19). Those 410 patients who did not achieve the goal of therapy, a diastolic blood pressure below 90 mmHg, were than rerandomized to an alternative monotherapy. The 102 nonresponders to the second drug were then given a combination of the first drug and the second. When the response rates for the various combinations were analyzed, those pairs that included a diuretic achieved a better response rate (69%) than combinations that did not include a diuretic (51%).

Although the numbers of patients who received the alpha-blocker prazosin along with another drug were small, they did about as well as the other combinations, but six of the eight terminations due to adverse drug reactions were in those combinations including prazosin. Three of the six were hypotensive reactions.

ALPHA-BLOCKERS IN RESISTANT PATIENTS

In the largest comparative controlled study published, one of five drugs or placebo was given, in a random order, to 238 patients whose diastolic pressure remained above 95 mmHg despite maximal doses of a diuretic and a beta blocker (20) (Figure 10-1). These latter two drugs were continued with-

TABLE 10-3. THE EFFECT OF DOXAZOSIN ADDED TO TRIPLE THERAPY

Variable	Run-in (4 wk)	Doxazosin (4 wk)	Washout (2 wk)
Supine systolic BP (mmHg)	161 ± 12	150 ± 12*	155 ± 17
diastolic BP (mmHG)	102 ± 4	93 ± 6†	95 ± 6
pulse rate (b/m)	69 ± 10	67 ± 8	64 ± 7
Standing systolic BP (mmHg)	157± 9	143 ± 12**	152 ± 16
diastolic BP (mmHg)	105 ± 5	96 ± 7**	100 ± 9
pulse rate (b/m)	74 ± 13	73 ± 10	71 ± 9

*$p < .09$.
**$p < .002$.
†$p < .001$.
BP = blood pressure.
(From Cappuccio and colleagues [22], with permission.)

out change in dose except in those allocated to labetalol who stopped the beta-blocker. All three drugs were given twice daily in these total doses (initial/maximal in mg): hydralazine (25/200), labetalol (400/3200), methyldopa (250/2000), minoxidil (5/40), and prazosin (2/20).

Of the five drugs, minoxidil was most effective but could only be used in 10 of the 35 patients who started it, mainly because of fluid retention that, because of the trial design, could not be handled as it likely would have been in clinical practice, by the addition of more diuretic. The other four agents were equally effective, but labetalol could be continued by only 9 of 41 patients because of side effects that may have been particularly bothersome because of the high doses of the drug used initially. Methyldopa could be continued by only 18 of 36 patients, again because of side effects. Hydralazine and prazosin could be continued in almost three-fourths of those given them. Thus, hydralazine and prazosin were equally effective and tolerated.

In a subsequent study of 93 patients uncontrolled on a thiazide and a beta-blocker, the same investigators randomly added nifedipine, prazosin, or hydralazine for 6 months (21). The three drugs were similar in regard to antihypertensive effect, withdrawal rate, and total number of side effects.

Another but smaller group of 10 patients with hypertension resistant to triple therapy (including an ACE inhibitor and a calcium antagonist) were given doxazosin in a median dose of 4 mg a day for 4 weeks after a 4-week run-in period and followed by a 2-week washout period (22). As seen in Table 10-3, the alpha-blocker induced a significant fall in both supine and standing blood pressure when added to the triple therapy.

SUMMARY AND CONCLUSIONS

Alpa-blockers are easy to add to other therapies including diuretics, beta-blockers, ACE inhibitors, and calcium antagonists. When added as the third or fourth drug to patients resistant to two or three, they lower the blood pressure further. Because of their different mode of inducing vasodilation, they are logical choices for patients not adequately controlled with other agents. Since the side effects of the newer agents are usually benign and since they possess unique abilities of improving lipids and insulin sensitivity and relieving the obstructive symptoms of prostatism, their use should continue to increase.

REFERENCES

1. Joint National Committee on Detection, Evaluation, and Treatment of High Blood Pressure. The fifth report of the Joint National Committee on Detection, Evaluation, and Treatment of High Blood Pressure (JNC V). *Arch Intern Med* 1993; 153:154–183.

2. Khoury AF, Kaplan NM. Alpha-blocker therapy of hypertension. An unfulfilled promise. *JAMA* 1991; 266:394–398.

3. Neaton JD, Grimm Jr RH, Prineas RJ, et al. Treatment of mild hypertension study. Final results. *JAMA* 1993; 270:713-724.

4. Kasiske BL, Ma JZ, Kalil RSN, Louis TA. Effects of antihypertensive therapy on serum lipids. *Ann Intern Med* 1995; 122:133–141.

5. Maheux P, Facchini F, Jeppesen J, et al. Changes in glucose, insulin, lipid, lipoprotein, and apoprotein concentrations and insulin action in doxazosin-treated patients with hypertension. *Am J Hypertens* 1994; 7:416–424.

6. Lepor H. α-Blockade for benign prostatic hyperplasia (BPH). *J Clin Endocrinol Metab* 1995; 80:750–753.

7. Lecerof H, Bornmyr S, Lilja B, et al. Acute effects of doxazosin and atenolol on smoking-induced peripheral vasoconstriction in hypertensive habitual smokers. *J Hypertens* 1990; 8(Suppl 5):S29–S33.

8. Fahrenbach MC, Yurgolevitch SM, Zmuda JM, Thompson PD. Effect of doxazosin or atenolol on exercise performance in physically active, hypertensive men. *Am J Cardiol* 1995; 75:258–263.

9. Bauer JH, Jones LB, Gaddy P. Effects of prazosin therapy on BP, renal function, and body fluid composition. *Arch Intern Med* 1984; 144:1196–1200.

10. Black HR, Chrysant SG, Curry CL, et al. Antihypertensive and metabolic effects of concomitant administration of terazosin and methyclothiazide for the treatment of essential hypertension. *J Clin Pharmacol* 1992; 32:351–359.

11. Searle M, Dathan R, Dean S, et al. Doxazosin in combination with atenolol in essential hypertension: a double-blind placebo-controlled multicentre trial. *Eur J Clin Pharmacol* 1990; 39:299–300.

12. Holtzman JL, Kaihlanen PM, Rider JA, et al. Concomitant administration of terazosin and atenolol for the treatment of essential hypertension. *Arch Intern Med* 1988; 148:539–543.

13. Brown MJ, Dickerson JEC. Synergism between alpha$_1$-blockade and angiotensin converting enzyme inhibition in essential hypertension. *J Hypertens* 1991; 9(Suppl 6):S362–S363.

14. Bainbridge AD, Meredith PA, Elliott HL. A clinical pharmacological assessment of doxazosin and enalapril in combination. *Br J Clin Pharmacol* 1993; 36:599–602.

15. Stokes GS, Johnston HJ, Okoro EO, et al. Comparative and combined efficacy of doxazosin and enalapril in hypertensive patients. *Clin Exp Hypertens* 1994; 16:709–727.

16. Elliott HL, Meredith PA, Campbell L, Reid JL. The combination of prazosin and verapamil in the treatment of essential hypertension. *Clin Pharmacol Ther* 1988; 43:554–560.

17. Donnelly R, Elliott HL, Meredith PA, et al. Combination of nifedipine and doxazosin in essential hypertension. *J Cardiovasc Pharmacol* 1992; 19:479–486.

18. Lenz ML, Pool JL, Laddu AR, et al. Combined terazosin and verapamil therapy in essential hypertension. Hemodynamic and pharmacokinetic interactions. *Am J Hypertens* 1995; 8:133–145.

19. Materson BJ, Reda DJ, Cushman WC, Henderson WG. Results of combination antihypertensive therapy after failure of each of the components. *J Hum Hypertens* 1995; 9: 791–796.

20. McAreavey D, Ramsey LE, Latham L, et al. "Third drug" trial: comparative study of antihypertensive agents added to treatment when blood pressure remains uncontrolled by a beta-blocker plus thiazide diuretic. *Br Med J* 1984; 288:106–111.

21. Ramsay LE, Parnell L, Waller PC. Comparison of nifedipine, prazosin and hydralazine added to treatment of hypertensive patients uncontrolled by thiazide diuretic plus beta-blocker. *Postgrad Med J* 1987; 63:99–103.

22. Cappuccio FP, Markandu ND, Whitcher F, MacGregor GA. Doxazosin in combination therapy for resistant hypertension [abstract]. *J Hypertens* 1994; 12(Suppl 3):S108.

Effects of Combination Therapy on the Heart

Franz H. Messerli

The heart has a dual role in hypertensive cardiovascular disease: Not only does it generate the force serving to sustain arterial pressure at its elevated level, but as a target organ it also suffers from the sustained increase in afterload (1). Antihypertensive therapy is prone to interact with both of these pathophysiological processes. The most common manifestation of hypertensive heart disease is left ventricular hypertrophy (LVH), arbitrarily defined as an increase in left ventricular mass exceeding certain established criteria. Although at first glance such an increase in muscle mass may be considered compensatory, numerous studies now attest to the fact that LVH distinctly and independently of blood pressure increases cardiovascular morbidity and mortality (2–5). Interestingly enough, hypertensive heart disease is usually accompanied by a blood pressure elevation severe enough to require two or more drugs to bring it under control. Thus a combination of two or more drugs is most commonly used in patients with hypertensive heart disease. In contrast, most studies dealing with the reduction of LVH were carried out by focusing on the effects of monotherapy on left ventricular mass. Most of what is known at the present with regard to combination therapy has, therefore, to be extrapolated from studies with monotherapy. It has to be borne in mind that these extrapolations, however provocative and suggestive clinically, may not always prove to be beneficial in terms of morbidity and mortality.

LEFT VENTRICULAR HYPERTROPHY

Several studies, meta-analyses and prospective have shown that ACE inhibitors are probably the most powerful monotherapeutic way to reduce LVH (5–7). Recently Schmieder and colleagues (8) performed a meta-analysis that only considered randomized studies comparing the effects of two or more therapies by assessing LVH and structure with blindly read echocardiograms. Out of more than 400 applications, only 391 clinical trials fulfilled these criteria. Similar to previous meta-analyses, the decrease in left ventricular mass was greater with active drug treatment than with placebo and was directly related to the pretreatment left ventricular mass, control of pressure, and duration of treatment. When the analysis was adjusted for the study duration, ACE inhibitors were most efficient in reducing LVH, followed by calcium channel blockers, the diuretics, and the beta-blockers (8). Indeed, some reports suggest that ACE inhibitors may lower blood pressure more than one would expect from their unloading properties alone. Calcium antagonists, as a class, seem slightly less potent in reducing LVH than the ACE inhibitors with heart rate-lowering agents possibly having a greater effect than the dihydropyridines. A lesser effect is assigned to the beta-blockers, the postsynaptic alpha-blockers, as well as the diuretics. Of note, however, is that recent findings in 690 men from the VA cooperative study (9) showed hydrochlorothiazide to be more efficacious than atenolol, captopril, diltiazem, prazosin, or clonidine. It must be emphasized, however, that with a few exceptions (10–12) there are no prospective, randomized, controlled trials comparing the effects of various antihypertensive drugs on left ventricular mass. Also, there is uncertainty as to what a drug-induced reduction of LVH exactly means in terms of morbidity and mortality.

There are no conclusive data that a reduction in LVH would confer a benefit that exceeded the one conferred by the reduction in arterial pressure per se. These drawbacks notwithstanding, it can be extrapolated that the combination of an ACE inhibitor with a calcium blocker ought to be particularly

TABLE 11-1. POSSIBLE SYNERGISM RESULTING FROM A COMBINATION OF A CALCIUM ANTAGONIST AND AN ACE INHIBITOR

	DHP-Calcium Antagonist	HRL-Calcium Antagonist	ACE Inhibitor
Kidneys			
↑Renal blood flow	Yes	Yes	Yes
↑Efferent vasodilation	Little	Yes	Yes
↑Afferent vasodilation	Yes	Yes	Yes
↓Microproteinuria	Little	Yes	Yes
"Renoprotection"	Unknown	Possible	Yes
Vascular Tree			
↓Endothelin-mediated vasoconstriction	Yes	Yes	No
↑Nitric oxide release	No	No	Yes
↑Arterial compliance	Yes	Yes	Yes
↓Vascular hypertrophy	Yes	Yers	Yes
↓Atherogenesis	Yes	Yes	Yes
Heart			
↓Left ventricular hypertrophy	Yes	Yes	Yes
↑Left ventricular filling	Yes	Yes	No
↑Contractility, unloading	Some	No	Yes
↑Coronary flow	Yes	Yes	Some
Secondary "cardioprotection"	No	Some	Yes

ACE = angiotensin-converting enzyme; DHP = dihydropyridine; HRL = heart rate lowering.

efficacious with regard to a reduction of LVH (Table 11-1). Because both of these drug classes have the potential to interfere with pathogenesis of LVH at a similar level, one can argue that this combination will reduce LVH more than one would expect from its blood pressure-lowering effects alone. Whether angiotensin receptor inhibitors, either in monotherapy or in combination, are as efficient as ACE inhibitors in reducing LVH remains undocumented at the present time. Most of the other commonly used combinations, such as diuretics plus beta-blockers, ACE inhibitors plus beta-blockers, as well as beta-blockers plus dihydropyridine calcium antagonists, are prone to reduce LVH in parallel with the fall in arterial pressure.

Is there any drug combination that should be avoided in patients with LVH? Drug classes that either stimulate the renin-angiotensin system or the sympathetic nervous system, or both, are less likely to reduce LVH than drug classes not stimulating these systems. The combination of an arteriolar vasodilator, such as hydralazine or minoxidil, with a diuretic should therefore probably not be used in an asymptomatic patient with LVH. Such a combination may also synergistically elicit hypokalemia, which could aggravate or trigger ventricular arrhythmias.

HYPERTENSION AND CORONARY ARTERY DISEASE

For a variety of pathophysiological reasons, the whole spectrum of coronary artery disease (microvascular to macrovascular, asymptomatic to symptomatic, silent ischemia to AMI) is very common in the patients with essential hypertension (13, 14). The two drug classes most commonly used to treat coronary artery disease are the calcium antagonists and the beta-blockers. It seems logical, therefore, to use a combination of these two drug classes in hypertensive patients who are suffering from coronary artery disease and require two or more drugs for lowering of arterial pressure. Indeed, fixed combinations of some dihydropyridine calcium antagonists and beta-blockers have been marketed outside the United States (15, 16). Of note, however, is that these combinations have been marketed for hypertension only and not for coronary artery disease. By and large, the combination of a heart rate-lowering calcium antagonist (verapamil, diltiazem) with a beta-blocker should be avoided because the two molecules could exert synergistic negative chronotropic and negative inotropic effects.

THE POSTMYOCARDIAL INFARCTION PATIENT

Numerous studies have documented that beta-blockers are the treatment of choice for preventing reinfarction in the patient who has suffered AMI (17). Similarly, ACE inhibitors have been shown to be beneficial in that they prevent remodeling (and thereby reduce the long-term risk of congestive heart failure), and reduce reinfarction rates and even sudden death (18). In contrast to beta-blockers and ACE inhibitors, the role of calcium antagonists in the postmyocardial infarction patient is less well established. In the Danish Verapamil Infarction Trial (DAVIT) II study (19), verapamil significantly reduced reinfarction rates when started 1 to 2 weeks after the acute event. Similarly, in the Multicenter Diltiazem Postinfarction Trial (MDPIT) study (20), diltiazem was shown to have some benefits in the patient with a non-Q-wave infarction. The effects of both verapamil and diltiazem were more pronounced in patients with hypertension (21) as well as in patients without congestive heart failure. It must be emphasized, however, that the fact that beta-blockers, heart rate-lowering calcium antagonists, and ACE inhibitors have some benefit in the post-myocardial infarction patient does by no means imply that their combination is as good as or even better than monotherapy. We therefore advise caution when using this combination for the prevention of reinfarction, although it seems reasonable to consider a low-dose combination of these agents in the patient who concomitantly is suffering from hypertension and needs combination therapy for blood pressure control.

HYPERTENSION, SYSTOLIC DYSFUNCTION, AND CONGESTIVE HEART FAILURE

Congestive heart failure is a common sequela for long-standing hypertension (22). It has been well documented that left ventricular systolic function declines with progression of hypertensive heart disease (23). Clearly, therefore, in the patient with systolic dysfunction, drugs that exert negative inotropic effects, such as some calcium antagonists and beta-blockers, should be used with restraint. It must be remembered, however, that low doses of beta-blockers have been shown to be beneficial, particularly in patients suffering from congestive heart failure as a result of dilated cardiomyopathy. Similarly, the new compound carvedilol was recently documented to improve morbidity and mortality in patients with congestive heart failure (24).

ACE inhibitors remain a cornerstone in the management of congestive heart failure and have been clearly shown to be of benefit early as well as late in the evolution of the disease. The standard therapy of congestive heart failure consists of a diuretic, digitalis, and an ACE inhibitor. Two of these drug classes are also commonly used to treat hypertension. In the PRAISE study (25), the addition of amlodipine was shown to have beneficial effects in patients with congestive heart failure from dilated cardiomyopathy. A reasonable combination to be used in such patients who are concomitantly suffering from hypertension would, therefore, be a diuretic, digitalis, an ACE inhibitor, and either amlodipine or dilevalol. Unlike amlodipine, which had no effect in patients with congestive heart failure caused by ischemic cardiomyopathy, carvedilol had equal benefits in patients with both dilated cardiomyopathy and ischemic cardiomyopathy.

HYPERTENSION, IMPAIRED LEFT VENTRICULAR FILLING, AND HYPERTROPHIC OBSTRUCTIVE CARDIOMYOPATHY

The most commonly used drugs to treat hypertrophic obstructive cardiomyopathy (HCOM) are the calcium antagonists and the beta-blockers. Both of these drug classes are commonly used in the treatment of hypertension and, therefore, can be combined in a patient concomitantly suffering from HCOM and hypertension. Of note, heart rate-lowering calcium antagonists may have a greater benefit than the dihydropyridines because the former prolong diastole and allow better left ventricular filling. HCOM may, therefore, be an indication for the combination of a heart rate-lowering calcium antagonist with a beta-blocker. This combination requires careful electrocardiographic monitoring since it may lead to an atrioventricular block or unmask sick sinus syndrome.

Left ventricular filling is also commonly impaired in patients with LVH and hypertensive heart disease (26–28). However, most often this impairment is asymptomatic and does not necessitate specific therapy. In the occasional patient who is suffering from dyspnea on exertion secondary to impaired filling, the addition of either a calcium antagonist or a beta-blocker to the current antihypertensive regimen should be sufficient. ACE inhibitors have been shown to improve LV filling inconsistently, when given for a prolonged period of time (29). In contrast to the findings with calcium antagonists and beta-blockers, which also have a direct effect on the early rapid filling phase, the effect by the ACE inhibitors seems to be solely mediated by their potential to improve ventricular compliance secondary to a reduction in LVH.

HYPERTENSION AND ARRHYTHMIAS

When treating coincidental arrhythmias in the hypertensive patient, one should remember that there are two drug classes that are electrophysiologically active and are commonly used to treat high blood pressure—the beta-blockers and the heart rate-lowering calcium antagonists. It seems logical, therefore, to consider either a heart rate-lowering calcium antagonist or a beta-blocker in the hypertensive patient who is concomitantly suffering from symptomatic arrhythmias and who needs additional therapy for lowering of arterial pressure, based on the electrophysiological indication or contraindication.

SUMMARY AND CONCLUSIONS

Much of what we know with regard to the effects of combination therapy on the heart is based on extrapolation from monotherapy. Although combination therapy is commonly used for the treatment of hypertension, its repercussions on the heart and specifically on hypertensive heart disease remain poorly documented. Given the fact that two drugs when used separately are beneficial in a disorder does not necessarily mean that their combination is equally or more beneficial. We therefore urge physicians to restrain the use of combination therapy primarily for the lowering of arterial pressure and only secondarily to consider concomitant pathophysiolical conditions associated with hypertensive heart disease.

REFERENCES

1. Messerli FH, Devereux RB. Left ventricular hypertrophy: good or evil? Proceedings of a symposium: left ventricular hypertrophy in essential hypertension—mechanisms and therapy. *Am J Med* 1983; 75(3A):1–3.

2. Kannel WB, Gordon T, Offutt D. Left ventricular hypertrophy by electrocardiogram. Prevalance, incidence and mortality in the Framingham study. *Ann Intern Med* 1969; 71:89–105.

3. Devereux RB, De Simone G, Koren MJ, et al. Left ventricular mass as a predictor of development of hypertension. *Am J Hypertens* 1991; 4:603S–607S.

4. Levy D, Garrison RJ, Savage DD, et al. Prognostic implications of echocardiographically determined left ventricular mass in the Framingham heart study. *N Engl J Med* 1990; 322:1561–1566.

5. Dahlöf B, Pennert K, Hansson L. Reversal of left ventricular hypertrophy in hypertensive patients. A meta-analysis of 109 treatment studies. *Am J Hypertens* 1992; 5:95–110.

6. Weidman BL, de Courten M, Eme P, Shaw S. Antihypertensive drug effects on left ventricular hypertrophy: meta-analysis considering duration of treatment [abstract]. *J Hypertens* 1994; 12 (Suppl 3):S140.

7. Cruickshank JM, Lewis J, Moore V, Dodd C. Reversibility of left ventricular hypertrophy by differing types of antihypertensive therapy. *J Hum Hypertens* 1992; 6(2):85–90.

8. Schmieder RE, Martus P, Klingbeil A. Reversal of left ventricular hypertrophy in essential hypertension. *JAMA* 1996; 275:1507–1513.

9. Gottdiener JS, Reda DJ, Williams DW, et al. Regression of left ventricular mass with monotherapy in mild-moderate hypertension: interaction of drug with systolic blood pressure, age, race and weight. *Circulation* 1994; 90 (Suppl):I-565.

10. Dahlöf B, Hansson L. Regression of left ventricular hypertrophy in previously untreated essential hypertension: different effects of enalapril and hydrochlorothiazide. *J Hypertens* 1992; 10:1513–1524.

11. Dahlöf B, Hansson L. The influence of antihypertensive therapy on the structural arteriolar changes in essential hypertension: different effects of enalapril and hydrochlorothiazide. *J Intern Med* 1993; 234:271–279.

12. Gottdiener J, Reda D, Notargiacomo A, et al. Comparison of monotherapy on LV mass regression in mild-to-moderate hypertension: echocardiographic results of a multicenter trial [abstract]. *J Am Coll Cardiol* 1991; 17(Suppl A):178A.

13. Kannel WB, Gordon T, Castelli WP, Margolis JR. Electrocardiographic left ventricular hypertrophy and risk of coronary heart disease. The Framingham study. *Ann Intern Med* 1970; 72:813–822.

14. Strauer BE. Left ventricular hypertrophy, myocardial blood flow and coronary reserve [review]. *Cardiology* 1992; 81:274–282.

15. Messerli FH. Combination therapy in essential hypertension. *Ann Intern Med* 1996; (submitted for publication).

16. Dahlöf B, Jönsson L, Borgholst O, et al. Improved antihypertensive efficacy of the felodipine-metoprolol extended-release tablet compared with each drug alone. *Blood Press* 1993; 1:37–45.

17. Yusuf S, Peto R, Lewis J, et al. Beta-blockade during and after myocardial infarction. An overview of the randomized trials. *Prog Cardiovasc Dis* 1985; 27:335–371.

18. Pfeffer MA, Braunwald E, Moye LA, et al. Effect of captopril on mortality and morbidity in patients with left ventricular dysfunction after myocardial infarction. Results of the survival and ventricular enlargement trial. The SAVE investigators. *N Engl J Med* 1992; 327:669–677.

19. The Danish Study Group on Verapamil in Myocardial Infarction. Effect of verapamil on mortality and major events after acute myocardial infarction. (The Danish Verapamil Infarction Trial II-DAVIT II). *Am J Cardiol* 1990; 66:779–785.

20. Moss AJ, Rubison M, Oakes D, et al. Effect of diltiazem on long-term outcome in post-infarction patients with a history of hypertension [abstract]. *Circulation* 1989; 80(Suppl II): II-268.

21. Messerli FH, Boden WE, Fischer Hansen J, Schechtman B. Heart rate lowering calcium antagonists (HRL-CA) in hypertensive post MI patients [abstract]. *JACC* 1996; 27(2):178A.

22. Kannel WB, Castelli WP, McNamara PM, et al. Role of blood pressure in the development of congestive heart failure. The Framingham study. *N Engl J Med* 1972; 287(16):781–787.

23. Grossman E, Oren S, Messerli FH. Left ventricular mass and cardiac function in patients with essential hypertension. *J Hum Hypertens* 1994; 8:417–421.

24. Carlson WD, Gilbert EM. Carvedilol. In: Messerli FH, ed. *Cardiovascular drug therapy*. 2nd ed. Philadelphia: W.B. Saunders, 1996: 583–600.

25. Frishman WH, Hershman D. Amlodipine. In: Messerli FH, ed. 1996: 1024–1040.

26. Smith VE, Schulman P, Karimeddini MK, et al. Rapid ventricular filling in left ventricular hypertrophy: II. Pathologic hypertrophy. *J Am Coll Cardiol* 1985; 5:869–874.

27. White WB, Schulman P, Karimeddini MK, Smith V-E. Regression of left ventricular mass is accompanied by improvement in rapid left ventricular filling following antihypertensive therapy with metoprolol. *Am Heart J* 1989; 117:145–150.

28. Wikstrand J. Left ventricular function in early primary hypertension. Functional consequences of cardiovascular structural changes. *Hypertension* 1984; 6(6 Part 2):III-108–III-116.

29. Opie LH. ACE inhibitors and the heart. In: *Angiotensin-converting enzyme inhibitors: scientific basis for clinical use*. 2nd ed. New York: Wiley-Liss, 1994: 94–97.

CHAPTER 12

Calcium Channel Blockade and/or ACE Inhibition for Prevention of Diabetic and Hypertensive Nephropathy

Prasad K. Kilaru and George L. Bakris

Diabetes is the most common cause of end-stage renal disease (ESRD) in the United States, accounting for 36% of new patients starting renal dialysis over the past decade (1, 2). Nephropathy develops in approximately 35% to 40% of all people with diabetes and is already present in 3% of patients with non-insulin dependent diabetes mellitus (NIDDM) at the time of diagnosis (3). Albuminuria and elevated arterial pressure are also present in all diabetic subjects destined to develop nephropathy (3–4). Once renal disease becomes apparent, reduction of both these markers slows nephropathy progression (5). Aggressive blood glucose control also preserves renal function prior to development of established renal disease (6).

Hypertension alone accounts for about 28% of all ESRD patients on dialysis (2, 7, 8). Hypertension also complicates the natural history of almost all types of nephropathy and may actually accelerate their progression (9, 10). Several studies document the effectiveness of blood pressure control in slowing the progression of nephropathy (11–14). The natural history in the pathogenesis of diabetic nephropathy is different from that of hypertensive nephropathy (Table 12-1).

ACE inhibitors and the nondihydropyridine class of calcium antagonists are known to reduce proteinuria and nephropathy progression to a greater extent than predicted by blood pressure reduction alone (15–18). The mechanisms by which these drug classes preserve renal function, independent of their blood pressure-lowering effects, is discussed.

PATHOPHYSIOLOGY

Both hemodynamic and metabolic factors play important roles in the pathogenesis of diabetic nephropathy. The fundamental vascular abnormality in patients with diabetes is disturbed vascular reactivity, which originates from altered endothelial cell function (19–21). Consequently, regulation

TABLE 12-1. DIFFERENCES IN THE NATURAL HISTORY OF DIABETIC AND HYPERTENSIVE RENAL DISEASE

	Diabetes	Hypertension
Autoregulation Preserved	No	Yes
Vascular reactivity	Increased	Unchanged
Mesangial volume (KW kidney)	Increased	Unchanged
Microalbuminuria predictive of ESRD	Yes	No
Intraglomerular pressure	Increased	Increased
Glomerular membrane permeability (albuminuria)	Increased*	Increased

*Note that permeability increases leakage of glycated albumin, which is toxic to cells. Also note that the changes indicated here are in the early stages of the disease and, in some cases, intraglomerular pressure is derived from animal models.
KW kidney = Kimmelstiel-Wilson kidney; ESRD = end-stage renal disease.

of intraglomerula pressure and membrane permeability in the nephron are altered. The nonhemodynamic pathophysiological changes that occur are as follows:

- increased advanced glycosylation end products
- increased concentration of local growth factors (insulinlike growth factor-1, platelet-derived growth factor, transformation growth factor-β, platelet-activating factor, endothelin, angiotensin II, etc.)
- increased glomerular membrane shunting of glycated albumin
- increased extracellular matrix proteins (type IV collagen, fibronectin, laminin, etc.)

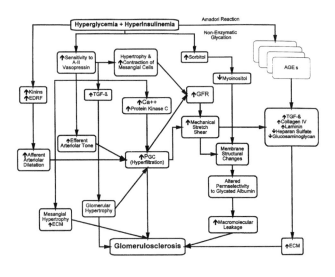

Figure 12-1. The interaction of hemodymanic and metabolic factors in the pathogenesis of renal disease from diabetes. AGEs = advanced glycosylation end products; TGF = transformation growth factor-β; ECM = extracellular matrix; P_{GC} = intraglomerular pressure; AII = angiotensin II; EDRF = endothelial-derived relaxing factor; GFR = glomerular filtration rate.

The interaction of both hemodynamic and nonhemodynamic factors is represented in Figure 12-1. A detailed discussion of how these changes affect nephropathy development are beyond the scope of this chapter; however, several comprehensive reviews cover this subject (22–25).

Of the markers that herald the presence of nephropathy in diabetes, persistent microalbuminuria (>30 mg/day, <300 mg/day) is one of the earliest. Capillary basement membrane thickening and expansion of the glomerular mesangium are the earliest morphological findings in diabetic nephropathy and relate directly to the genesis of microalbuminuria (26, 27). Moreover, mesangial expansion is the *earliest* morphological change associated with loss of renal function (26, 27).

Microalbuminuria has clearly different prognostic implications for nephropathy development in the diabetic compared to nondiabetic hypertensive subject (24, 28). This is postulated to be due to glycation of albumin in association with hyperglycemia. Glycation transforms albumin into a cellular toxin (24, 29, 30). Glycated albumin consequently stimulates production of reactive oxygen species by cells, and, hence, additional cell injury. The reader is referred to a recent review on this topic (24). The effects of ACE inhibitors and calcium channel blockers on these and related changes in the kidney are the focus of this chapter.

ACE Inhibition

The proposed actions of the ACE inhibitors within the kidney are as follows:

- reduce intraglomerular pressure
- improve glomerular permeability
- inhibit glomerular hypertrophy
- prevent glomerulosclerosis
- reduce mesangial matrix expansion
- reduce interstitial fibrosis
- inhibit procollagen formation
- increase natriuresis
- reduce proteinuria
- improve survival

Early studies with the combination of hydrochlorthiazide, hydralazine, and reserpine were unable to reduce the intraglomerular hypertension despite successfully reducing the systemic blood pressure in experimental animals (31). This failure to reduce glomerular hypertension was manifested by increases in proteinuria and glomerular scarring comparable to those seen in the untreated group. However, recent studies using 24-hour blood pressure monitoring in the same animal model demonstrate similar protection by both ACE inhibitors and triple therapy (32). This suggests that ACE inhibitors may not be different when blood pressure is lowered to certain levels. However, it supports the concept that unless glomerular capillary hypertension is corrected, control of systemic blood pressure alone is insufficient to prevent progression of renal injury.

In several other experimental models, ACE inhibitors clearly slow morphological progression of diabetic renal disease and prevent the development of glomerulosclerosis (25, 33–36). ACE inhibitors also reduce microalbuminuria and blunt the progression of albuminuria (25, 33–36). In addition to the reduction in intraglomerular pressure (P_{GC}), there is also evidence that mesangial matrix expansion is slowed when shunting of glycated albumin through the glomerular capillary membrane pores is reduced (24, 36–38).

In vitro experiments demonstrate that ACE inhibitors under normal as well as hyperglycemic conditions attenuate angiotensin II-induced increases in cell size and growth (39). They also attenuate hyperglycemia-induced increases of matrix proteins such as laminin and fibronectin, as well as blunt reductions of heparan sulfate and glucosaminoglycan (40, 41). Thus, ACE inhibitors may prevent mesangial matrix expansion and ultimately glomerulosclerosis through actions independent of blood pressure reduction. It should be noted, however, that many of the studies evaluating matrix protein synthesis did not have appropriate control groups for blood pressure reduction. Hence, it is not entirely clear whether the effects of these agents are indeed independent of arterial pressure reduction.

Elevated expression of transforming growth factor-beta (TGF-β) is present in a number of experimental glomerular diseases, including diabetic nephropathy (42). Angiotensin II (AII) is one of the growth factors that stimulates gene expression of TGF-β, fibronectin, and laminin. Moreover, studies in animal models of glomerulonephritis as well as diabetic nephropathy strongly implicate TGF-β in the pathogenesis of mesangial matrix buildup (42). Since AII plays an important role in the induction of TGF-β, ACE inhibitors are expected to reduce the TGF-β levels (43). The AT_1 receptor antagonist TCV-116 reduces gene expression of fibronectin; types I, III, and IV collagen; and laminin in the left ventricle, aorta, and the mesenteric artery of the rat (44). This is also evidenced by the in vivo effects of alacepril, an ACE inhibitor, and SC-52458, an angiotensin (AT_1) receptor antagonist. Both agents also reduced mRNA levels of TGF-β in spontaneously hypertensive rats (43).

HUMAN STUDIES

Hypertensive Nondiabetic Studies

In various studies of nondiabetic patients with different etiologies of nephropathy, ACE inhibitors have consistently reduced proteinuria and progression of nephropathy (45–48). In a retrospective study, Mann and colleagues (47) noted that three times more people were on dialysis at the end of 2 years of blood pressure treatment with non-ACE-inhibiting agents than those who received ACE inhibitors. In a prospective, randomized, open-label study over a 26-month period, enalapril slowed progression of nondiabetic renal disease (48). A 7-year follow-up of these patients demonstrated that 12 of the 35 patients (34%) in the original enalapril group were alive without renal replacement therapy versus 5 of the 35 patients (14%) in the control group. This difference of 20% in favor of enalapril was statistically significant ($p = .05$; 95% confidence limits, 0.5% to 39.5%) (49).

These observations of ACE inhibitors on preservation of renal function are further bolstered by a recent meta-analysis of all studies involving hypertensive patients and renal disease progression. Patients with chronic renal failure who were treated with ACE inhibitors had a significantly reduced progression of renal disease compared to conventional antihypertensive therapy (50).

Diabetic Studies

Several studies document that ACE inhibitors are more effective in decreasing albuminuria or proteinuria and improving renal survival in diabetic nephropathy than other antihypertensives (17, 18, 22, 24, 25, 50–53). In a randomized, controlled trial, patients with overt nephropathy from insulin-dependent diabetes mellitus were given either captopril or placebo for a median period of 2.7 years (17). Captopril treatment doubled the time required to reach dialysis compared to the blood pressure-lowering therapies. Moreover, a subgroup analysis of patients with nephrotic-range proteinurian at study entry demonstrated that only those who had sustained reductions in proteinuria had a slowed progression of renal disease (53). The remission rate was 16.7% in the captopril group compared to 1.5% in the placebo group. One important factor that may account for this difference is the degree of blood pressure reduction. The captopril group had significantly lower blood pressures (126/81 ± 8/8 mmHg), with a greater reduction from baseline compared to the placebo group (140/85 ±13/8 mmHg). This difference in blood pressure reduction may account for the observed differences in remission rates.

In a recent meta-analysis of 104 published studies involving more than 2,000 patients, Weidmann and colleagues (54) demonstrate that ACE inhibitors reduce proteinuria by 37% and nonhydropyridine calcium channel blockers by 33%, whereas short-acting nifedipine actually increases proteinuria by 5%. These observations could not be accounted for by differences in the blood pressure reduction between treatment groups. The fastest rate of decline in renal function was also noted in the nifedipine studies with a decline in glomerular filtration rate (GFR) of 48% per year, compared to 1% per year for ACE inhibitors, 8% for placebo, and 9% for the combination of diuretics and β-blockers. ACE inhibitors were also the only drugs that reduced proteinuria, even if no reduction in blood pressure was achieved. Similar observations were derived by Maki and associates (50). In this meta-analysis, 14 randomized, controlled trials with ACE inhibitors resulted in a greater decrease in proteinuria and preservation of GFR compared to other agents (50). Moreover, these authors noted that for each 10-mmHg reduction in blood pressure there was an additional decrease in proteinuria, but ACE inhibitors and nonhydrophridine calcium channel blockers were associated with additional declines in proteinuria independent of blood pressure changes and diabetes.

ACE inhibitors also delay progression of diabetic renal disease and blunt increases in microalbuminuria when given to normotensive individuals for as long as 7 years (51, 52, 55). However, based on current knowledge, ACE inhibitors should only be given to normotensive patients with microalbuminuria and insulin-dependent diabetes mellitus, not to all diabetic subjects.

CALCIUM CHANNEL BLOCKADE

Calcium channel blockers block calcium entry into the cell by inhibiting one of the more than seven different calcium channels present on cells. Calcium channels have different effects on the vasculature, heart, and nerves, depending on which is stimulated or inhibited. Moreover, not all cells contain all calcium channels, thus partially explaining the diversity of actions by this class of drugs.

Calcium channel blockers have a significantly diverse therapeutic spectrum of activity. Based on their actions, it is convenient to divide them into dihydropyridine and nondihydropyridine groups. Their proposed intrarenal effects are as follows:

- improve glomerular permeability
- reduce glomerulosclerosis
- reduce formation of oxygen free radicals
- prevent glomerular hypertrophy
- increase natriuresis
- reduce platelet aggregation
- reduce intracellular calcium accumulation
- reduce renal hypermetabolism
- reduce proteinuria

In the kidney their effects on the efferent arteriole differ, but they all dilate the afferent arteriole (56–58). The dihydropyridine calcium channel blockers (e.g., nifedipine) have no effect on the efferent arterioles, whereas the nondihydropyridine group (e.g., diltiazem, verapamil, etc.) partially dilate these arterioles (57, 58). This divergent effect is explained by the lack of dihydropyridine calcium channels on the efferent arteriole (59). Since this efferent arteriolar dilatation is minimal in the face of afferent dilatation, systemic blood pressure needs to be significantly lowered to reduce intraglomerular pressure with all types of calcium channel blockers. Thus, the disparate results on proteinuria and preservation of renal function obtained from within this class of agents cannot be explained on the basis of hemodynamic differences alone.

Cell/Animal Studies

Nondihydropyridine calcium channel blockers and ACE inhibitors reduce proteinuria and slow the progression of glomerulosclerosis in animal models of diabetes (25, 50, 54). In the remnant kidney model, verapamil was found effective in protecting the kidney even without any reduction in the systemic or glomerular capillary pressure. This protection correlated with decreased calcium salt deposition (60, 61). However, this benefit is only seen if verapamil is started before the glomeruli show compensatory hypertrophy (62).

Dworkin and colleagues (63) studied the effect of enalapril, nifedipine, or no therapy in rats with a 5/6 nephrectomy. Both nifedipine and enalapril reduced the systemic blood pressure as well as the severity of the glomerular injury. While enalapril reduced the intraglomerular pressure, nifedipine failed to do so. Despite this failure, kidney weight, glomerular volume, and glomerular capillary radius were smaller in the nifedipine group, indicating that compensatory hypertrophy was lessened by the nifedipine therapy. The prevalence of glomerular sclerosis was also the lowest in the nifedipine group, indicating that calcium channel blockers act by different mechanisms in protecting the kidney in hypertension. It should also be noted that dihydropyridines are not uniformly protective at a given blood pressure. This has as much to do with the animal studied as with the level of blood pressure achieved. This is evidenced by a recent report from the same group with amlodipine (64). In this study, a deoxycorticosterone acetate (DOCA) salt as well as a uninephrectomized, spontaneously hypertensive rat model of hypertension were used. Amlodipine in these models did not reduce glomerular pressure, proteinuria, or prevalence of glomerulosclerosis.

Since calcium channel blockers preferentially dilate the afferent arterioles, normalization of systemic blood pressure is essential to shield the glomeruli from its deleterious effects. A comparison of nifedipine and enalapril in a remnant rat kidney model illustrates this concept. Enalapril was able to provide proportional protection to the reduction of the blood pressure, whereas nifedipine did not protect against scarring of the nephron (65). This study further demonstrates that to equal the degree of protection afforded to the kidney with ACE inhibitors at a blood pressure of 130/80 mmHg, with nifedipine the pressure should be reduced to 100/60 mmHg (65). The renal autoregulatory indices were the highest for the nifedipine group and were close to or better than the control group in the enalapril group. These authors propose that nifedipine blocks renal autoregulation, hence eliminating a key physiological protective mechanism of the kidney against high pressures. Interestingly, renal autoregulation is not totally inhibited by either verapamil or diltiazem (35, 57, 66). This may account for some of their beneficial effects on the kidney.

Studies with nondihydropyridine calcium channel blockers demonstrate an ability to blunt declines in the synthesis of mesangial matrix proteins like heparan sulfate and glucosaminoglycan in a fashion similar to ACE inhibitors (67). This phenomenon may explain why nondihydropyridine calcium channel blockers are consistently more renoprotective than the dihydropyridines. Verapamil, another nondihydropyridine calcium channel blocker, has also been shown to blunt mesangial volume expansion in diabetic animal models (68).

Human Studies

In a retrospective study of African-American patients with moderate renal insufficiency, Brazy and Fitzwilliam (14) document that maintenance of diastolic blood pressure below 90 mmHg was associated with a 40% slower progression of renal disease when compared to those with diastolic pressures greater than 90 mmHg. Interestingly, those treated with calcium channel blockers or minoxidil had the slowest rates of decline. These observations have been recently confirmed in a 6-year follow-up of a randomized, prospective, open-label study involving 29 African-American patients with NIDDM-associated nephropathy (69). This study demonstrates that those randomized to either verapamil SR or diltiazem SR had a 65% slower rate of decline in glomerular filtration rate and an 83% greater reduction in proteinuria compared to those who received atenolol. All subjects received diuretics.

Unfortunately, there are very few long-term studies (i.e., greater than 2 years duration) that examine the effects of calcium channel blockers on progression of diabetic nephropathy. Only three well-constructed studies exist: one with nondihydropyridine calcium channel blockers and two others with the dihydropyridine calcium channel blockers nifedipine and amlodipine. In a recent 6-year follow-up study, 52 patients with nephropathy from NIDDM were randomized to receive either an ACE inhibitor or a nondihydropyridine calcium channel blocker (verapamil SR or dilitiazem SR) and atenolol. The blood pressure goal was less than 140/90 mmHg. At the end of a mean follow-up period of 63 months, there was no significant difference in the rate of decline in GFR between the ACE inhibitor and nondihydropyridine calcium channel blocker groups. Both, however, were approximately 60% slower than the atenolol group (18). In the second study (70), the Melbourne Diabetes Study Group compared the effects of nifedipine to perindopril on progression of nephropathy in a combined group of NIDDM and insulin-dependent diabetic patients. This group, while initially reporting no difference in proteinuria reduction between either group at 1 year, reported no change from baseline with nifedipine at 2 years. This result occurred in spite of sustained blood pressure reductions. No data are as yet available on the progression of nephropathy. This proteinuria result is predictable, since nifedipine does not alter glomerular membrane pore shunting of albumin or charge selectivity (71). The last of these studies (72) compares the effects of cilazapril and amlodipine on kidney function in 44 hypertensive patients with NIDDM over a 3-year period. Twenty-six of 44 patients were normalbuminuric and 18 had microalbuminuria. In the microalbuminuric high-risk group, the rate of decline in GFR was not significantly different between the two groups, both of which averaged a decline of 2.2 ml/minute/year/1.73 m^2.

COMBINATION THERAPY

Given that ACE inhibitors and calcium channel blockers yield similar effects on blood pressure reduction through different and potentially complementary mechanisms, combining them may have potentially beneficial effects on the kidney. This is exemplified when nifedipine was combined with enalapril and found to be more efficacious in reducing proteinuria and preventing development of glomerulosclerosis than nifedipine alone (73). It was not significantly better, however, than enalapril alone.

Cell/Animal Studies

Recent studies in a two-kidney-1 clip hypertensive rat model demonstrated that nitrendipine alone was not able to afford any protection against glomerulosclerosis (74). However, when combined with enalapril there was marked preservation of the nonclipped kidney. Unfortunately, it is difficult to assess the true effect of combination therapy on renal function, since blood pressure was significantly lower in the combined group.

The effects of combination therapy have also been assessed in uninephrectomized, alloxan-induced diabetic beagle dogs. Animals were randomized to receive either lisinopril, a diltiazemlike calcium antagonist, TA-3090, or a combination of both in lower doses so as to achieve the same level of blood pressure reduction (36). Lisinopril-treated dogs lowered their P_{GC} to that of the nondiabetic control dogs. Those treated with TA-3090 showed no reduction in P_{GC}. Despite this variation in P_{GC}, both treatments decreased glomerular hypertrophy as well as proteinuria and mesangial matrix expansion. Combination therapy attenuated increases in proteinuria to a greater degree than either agent alone. This occurred at similar levels of blood pressure reduction. There was not additive effect on mesangial matrix expansion, however, with combination therapy.

Lastly, the effects of verapamil alone or in combination with an ACE inhibitor were assessed in stroke-prone, spontaneously hypertensive rats (68). The goal of this study was to ascertain whether these agents provide protection against development of glomerulosclerosis in the absence of blood pressure reduction. This study demonstrated that the combination of verapamil and trandolopril reduced proteinuria and glomerulosclerosis to a greater extent than either agent alone. This observation occurred in the absence of any reduction in arterial pressure.

Human Studies

In 1990 it was first demonstrated that diltiazem and lisinopril had similar antiproteinuric effects with comparable blood pressure control (75). Thus, it would be predicted that the combination of these two agents may have additive antiproteinuric effects at similar levels of blood pressure reduction. An in-depth review of the hormonal and antiproteinuric response to combination therapy is beyond the scope of this chapter; however, the reader is referred to a recent review of this topic (76).

ACE inhibitors and calcium channel blockers do not interfere with each others' antihypertensive actions; moreover, their actions are synergistic (77). Such combinations may also reduce the adverse reactions associated with higher doses of either agent alone. An example of this is edema associated with nifedipine use, which disappeared in 3 out of 4 patients when an ACE inhibitor was added (78). In the same study, the combination lowered blood pressure more than monotherapy with either captopril or nifedipine alone. However, there were no significant differences in plasma renin activity or urinary aldosterone levels among the treatment groups.

While there are many studies that assess the effects of fixed-dose combinations of ACE inhibitors and calcium channel blockers on blood pressure lowering, there are only two studies that assess their effects on progression of renal disease. Both these studies are in patients with NIDDM-associated nephropathy. In the first, the combination of verapamil and lisinopril was given to 8 patients who were assessed after 1 and 6 years (18, 79). In this study, while treatment with the combination yielded blood pressure reductions comparable to either agent alone, the combination group had substantially lower amounts of proteinuria and the slowest rate of decline in GFR. Moreover, they had the lowest side effect profile. In the second study, patients with NIDDM nephropathy were randomized to either the combination of diltiazem and lisinopril or either agent alone, and were followed for 1 year. Subjects on combination therapy had the greatest reduction in proteinuria and the lowest side effect profile both in terms of edema and hyperkalemia (80).

SUMMARY AND CONCLUSIONS

In diabetic renal disease it is critically important to reduce albuminuria and keep blood pressure reduced to <130/80 mmHg (81). ACE inhibitors have shown clear superiority as initial antihypertensive therapy in this group as long as serum creatinine is less than 2.5 mg/dl. There is little experience on renal disease progression in patients with serum creatinines above this level. Addition of a nondihydropyridine calcium channel blocker to an ACE inhibitor shows a significant increase in the efficacy of blood pressure reduction as well as further lowering of proteinuria, this with decreased side effect profiles compared to either agent alone. There is little experience with dihydropyridine calcium channel blockers and ACE inhibitors in this group. Thus, this combination should be reserved for the recalcitrant hypertensive subject.

In hypertensive renal disease, the level of blood pressure reduction correlates with the degree of antiproteinuric effect of a given antihypertensive agent. The possible exceptions are the dihydropyridine calcium antagonists. Reductions in albuminuria, while associated with reduced cardiovascular mortality, have not been shown to affect renal mortality. Combinations of ACE inhibitors and calcium channel blockers have a clear role in this group if blood pressure cannot be controlled with a single agent. Moreover, fixed-dose combinations such as amlodipine-benazapril, verapamil/trandolapril, and others are well tolerated with minimal side effects.

REFERENCES

1. National Diabetes Fact Sheet. (National estimates for release on November 3, 1995.) Released by US CDC and available at http://www.cdc.gov/nccdphp/ddt/facts.htm#lt_comp.

2. Geiss LS, Herman WH, Goldschmid MG, et al. Surveillance for diabetes mellitus—United States 1980–1988. *MMWR* 1993; 42:1–20.

3. Gall MA, Rossing P, Slott P, et al. Prevalence of micro- and macroalbuminuria, arterial hypertension, retinopathy and large vessel disease in European type 2 (non-insulin dependent) diabetic patients. *Diabetalogia* 1991; 34:655–661.

4. Mogensen CE. Diabetes mellitus and the kidney. *Kidney Int* 1982; 21(5): 673–675.

5. Bakris GL. Blood pressure control and progression of diabetic nephropathy: are all drugs created equal? *Kidney: a current survey of world literature*. 1994; 3:61–62.

6. Barbosa J, Steffes MW, Sutherland DE, et al. Effect of glycemic control on early diabetic renal lesions. A 5-year randomized controlled clinical trial of insulin-dependent diabetic kidney transplant recipients. *JAMA* 1994; 272(8):600–666.

7. Whelton PK, Perneger TV, Brancati FL, et al. Epidemiology of blood pressure-related renal disease. *J Hypertens* 1992; 10 (Suppl 7):S77–S84.

8. Perneger TV, Whelton PK, Klag MJ, Rossiter KA. Diagnosis of hypertensive end-stage renal disease: effect of patient's race. *Am J Epidemiol* 1995; 141:10–15.

9. Sauter ER, Bakris GL. Effects of enalapril on urinary protein excretion in patients with idiopathic membranous nephropathy. *J Clin Pharmacol* 1990; 30: 155–158.

10. Rambausek M, Rhein C, Jaeger T, et al. Hypertension in chronic idiopathic glomerulonephritis: analysis of 311 biopsied patients. *Eur J Clin Invest* 1989; 19:176–180.

11. Eergstrom J, Alverstrand A, Bucht H, et al. Progression of chronic renal failure is retarded by more clinical follow-ups and better blood pressure control. *Clin Nephrol* 1986; 25:1–6.

12. Payton CD, McLay A, Boulton-Jones JM. Progressive IgA nephropathy: the role of hypertension. *Nephrol Dial Transplant* 1988; 2:138–142.

13. Alverstrand A, Guiterrez A, Bucht H, et al. Reduction of blood pressure retards the progression of chronic renal failure in man. *Nephrol Dial Transplant* 1988: 3:624–631.

14. Brazy PC, Fitzwilliam JF. Progressive renal disease: role of race and antihypertensive medications. *Kidney Int* 1990; 37(4):1113–1119.

15. Viberti G, Mogensen CE, Groop LC, Pauls JF. Effect of captopril on progression to clinical proteinuria in patients with insulin-dependent diabetes mellitus and micro-albuminuria. European Microalbuminuria Captopril Study Group. *JAMA* 1994; 271(4):275–279.

16. Slataper R, Vicknair N, Sadler R, Bakris GL. Comparative effects of different antihypertensive treatments on progression of diabetic renal disease. *Arch Intern Med* 1993; 153(8):973–980.

17. Lewis EJ, Hunsicker LG, Bain RP, Rhode RD. The effect of angiotensin-converting enzyme-inhibition on diabetic nephropathy. *N Engl J Med* 1993; 329:1456–1462.

18. Bakris GL, Copley JB, Vicknair N, Sadler R, Leurgans S. Calcium channel blockers versus other antihypertensive therapies on progression of NIDDM associated nephropathy: results of a six year study. *Kidnet Int* 1996; 50:1641–1650.

19. Komers R, Allen TJ, Cooper ME. Role of endothelium-derived nitric oxide in the pathogenesis of the renal hemodynamic changes of experimental diabetes. *Diabetes* 1994; 43(10):1190–1197.

20. Jaffa AA, Rust PF, Mayfield RK. Kinin, a mediator of diabetes-induced glomerular hyperfiltration. *Diabetes* 1995; 44(2):156–160.

21. Hutchison FN, Cui X, Webster SK. The antiproteinuric action of angiotensin converting enzyme is dependent on kinin. *J Am Soc Nephrol* 1995; 6:1216–1222.

22. Bakris GL. Abnormalities of calcium and the diabetic hypertensive patient: implications for renal preservation. In: Epstein M, ed. *Calcium antagonists in clinical medicine.* Philadelphia: Hanley & Belfus, 1992: 367–389.

23. Bakris GL, Williams B. ACE inhibitors and calcium antagonists alone or combined: Is there a difference on progression of diabetic renal disease? *Hypertension* 1995; 13(Suppl 2): S95–S101.

24. Bakris GL. Microalbuminuria: prognostic implications. *Curr Opin Nephrol Hypertens* 1996:5(3):219–223.

25. Bakris GL. Hyerptension in diabetic patients: an overview of interventional studies to preserve renal function. *Am J Hypertens* 1993; 6:140S–147S.

26. Mauer SM, Steffes MW, Ellis EM, et al. Structural functional relationship in diabetic nephropathy. *J Clin Invest* 1984; 74:1143–1155.

27. Steffes MW, Osterby R, Chavers B, Mauer SM. Mesangial expansion as a central mechanism for loss of kidney function in diabetic patients. *Diabetes* 1989; 39:1077–1081.

28. Kilaru P, Bakris GL. Microalbuminuria and progressive renal disease *J Hum Hypertens* 1994; 8:809–817.

29. Cohen M, Ziyadeh FN. Amadori glucose adducts modulate mesangial cell growth and collagen gene expression. *Kidney Int* 1994; 45:475–484.

30. Cohen MP, Hud E, Wu VY, Ziyadeh FN. Glycated albumin modified by Amadori adducts modulates aortic endothelial cell biology. *Mol Cell Biochem* 1995; 143(1):73–79.

31. Anderson S, Rennke HG, Brenner BM. Therapeutic advantage of converting enzyme inhibitors in arresting progressive renal disease associated with systemic hypertension in the rat. *J Clin Invest* 1986; 77(6):1993–2000.

32. Griffin KA, Picken M, Bidani AK. Radiotelemetric BP monitoring, antihypertensives and glomeruloprotection in remnant kidney model. *Kidney Int* 1994; 46(4):1010–1018.

33. Anderson S, Rennke HG, Garcia DL, et al. Short and long-term effects of antihypertensive therapy in the diabetic rat. *Kidney Int* 1989; 36:526–536.

34. Anderson S, Rennke HG, Brenner BM. Nifedipine versus fosinopril in uninephrectomized diabetic rats. *Kidney Int* 1992; 41:891–897.

35. Brown S, Walton C, Crawford P, Bakris GL. Comparative renal hemodynamic effects of an ACE-inhibitor or calcium antagonist on progression of diabetic nephropathy in the dog. *Kidney Int* 1993; 43:1210–1218.

36. Gaber L, Walton C, Brown S, Bakris GL. Effect of antihypertensive treatments on morphologic progression of diabetic nephropathy in uninephrectomized dogs. *Kidney Int* 1994; 46:161–169.

37. Myers BD. Pathophysiology of proteinuria in diabetic glomerular disease. *J Hypertens* 1990; 8(Suppl 1):S41–S46.

38. Scandling JD, Myers BD. Glomerular size selectivity and microalbuminuria in early diabetic glomerular disease. *Kidney Int* 1992; 41:840–846.

39. Bakris GL, Bhandaru S, Akerstrom V, Re RN. ACE inhibitor-mediated attenuation of mesangial cell growth: a role of endothelin. *Am J Hypertens* 1994; 7(7):583–590.

40. Reddi AS, Ramamurthi R, Miller M, et al. Enalapril improves albuminuria by preventing glomerular loss of heparan sulfate in diabetic rats. *Biochem Med Metab Biol* 1991; 45(1):119–131.

41. Nakamura T, Takahashi T, Fukui M, et al. Enalapril attenuates increased gene expression of extracellular matrix components in diabetic rats. *J Am Soc Nephrol* 1995; 5(7):1492–1497.

42. Yamamoto T, Nakamura T, Noble NA, et al. Expression of transforming growth factor-β is elevated in human and experimental diabetic nephropathy. *Proc Natl Acad Sci USA* 1993; 90(5):1814–1818.

43. Ohta K, Kim S, Hamaguchi A, et al. Role of angiotensin II in extracellular matrix and transforming growth factor-β expression in hypertensive rats. *Eur J Pharmacol* 1994; 269(1):115–119.

44. Kim S, Ohta K, Hamaguchi A, et al. Angiogensin II type I receptor antagonist inhibits the gene expression of transforming growth factor-β and extracellular matrix in cardiac and vascular tissues of hypertensive rats. *J Pharmacol Exp Ther* 1995; 273(1):509–515.

45. Kloke HJ, Wetzels JF, van Hamersvelt HW, et al. Effects of nitrendipine and cilazapril on renal hemodynamics and albuminuria in hypertensive patients with chronic renal failure. *J Cardiovasc Pharmacol* 1990; 16(6):924–930.

46. Zucchelli P, Zuccala A, Borghi M, et al. Long term comparison between captopril and nifedipine in the progression of renal insufficiency. *Kidney Int* 1992; 42:452–458.

47. Mann JF, Reisch C, Ritz E. Use of angiotensin-converting enzyme inhibitors for the preservation of kidney function. A retrospective study. *Nephron* 1990; 55(Suppl 1):38–44.

48. Kamper AL, Strandgaard S, Leyssac PP. Effect of enalapril on the progression of chronic renal failure. A randomized controlled trial. *Am J Hypertens* 1992; 5(7):423–430.

49. Kamper AL, Strandgaard S, Leyssac PP. Late outcome of a controlled trial of enalapril treatment in progressive chronic renal failure. Hard end-points and influence of proteinuria. *Nephrol Dial Transplant* 1995; 10(7):1182–1188.

50. Maki DD, Ma JZ, Louis TA, Kasiske BL. Long-term effects of antihypertensive agents on proteinuria and renal function. *Arch Intern Med* 1995; 155:1073–1080.

51. Ravid M, Lang R, Radimani R, Lishner M. Long term renoprotective effect of angiotensin-converting enzyme inhibition in noninsulin dependent diabetes mellitus: a 7 year follow-up study. *Arch Intern Med* 1996; 156:286–289.

52. Sano T, Kawamura T, Matsumae H, et al. Effects of long-term enalapril treatment on persistent microalbuminuria in well-controlled hypertensive and normotensive NIDDM patients. *Diabetes Care* 1994; 17(5):420–424.

53. Herbert LA, Bain RP, Verme D, et al. Remission of nephrotic range proteinuria in type I diabetes. Collaborative study group. *Kidney Int* 1994; 46(6):1688–1693.

54. Weidmann P, Schneider M, Bohlen L, et al. Therapeutic efficacy of different antihypertensive drugs in human diabetic nephropathy: an updated meta-analysis. *Nephrol Dial Transplant* 1995; 10(Suppl 9):39–45.

55. Slataper R, Vicknair N, Sadler R, Bakris GL. ACE inhibition normalizes renal size and mircoalbuminuria in normotensive insulin dependent diabetic patients. *J Diabetes Complications* 1994; 8:2–6.

56. Anderson S. Renal hemodynamics of calcium antagonists in rats with reduced renal mass. *Hypertension* 1991; 17:288–295.

57. Carmines PR, Navar LG. Disparate effects of CA channel blockade on afferent and efferent arteriolar response to Ang II. *Am J Physiol* 1989; 256(6 Part 2):F1015–F1020.

58. Conger JD, Falk SA. KCl and angiotensin responses in isolated rat renal artrioles: effects of diltiazem and low-calcium medium. *Am J Physiol* 1993; 264(1 Part 2):F134–F140.

59. Carmines P, Fowler BC, Bell PD. Segmentally distinct effects of depolarization on intracellular [Ca++] in renal arterioles. *Am J Physiol* 1993; 265:F677–F685.

60. Harris DC, Hammond WS, Burke TJ, Schrier RW. Verapamil protects against progression of experimental chronic renal failure. *Kidney Int* 1987; 31(1):41–46.

61. Pelayo JC, Harris DC, Shanley PF, et al. Glomerular hemodynamic adaptations in remnant nephrons: effects of verapamil. *Am J Physiol* 1988; 254 (3 Part 2):F425–F431.

62. Brunner FP, Thiel G, Hermle M, et al. Long-term enalapril and verapamil in rats with reduced renal mass. *Kidney Int* 1989; 36(6):969–977.

63. Dworkin LD, Benstein JA, Parker M, et al. Calcium antagonists and converting enzyme inhibitors reduce renal injury by different mechanisms. *Kidney Int* 1993; 43:808–814.

64. Dworkin L, Tolbert E, Recht PA, et al. Effects of amlodipine on glomerular filtration, growth and injury in experimental hypertension. *Hypertension* 1996; 27:245–250.

65. Griffin KA, Picken MM, Bidani AK. Deleterious effects of calcium channel blockade on pressure transmission and glomerular injury in rat remnant kidneys. *J Clin Inves* 1995: 96:793–800.

66. Loutzenhiser R, Epstein M, Horton C. Inhibition by diltiazem of pressure-induced afferent vasoconstriction in the isolated perfused rat kidney. *Am J Cardiol* 1987; 59:72A–75A.

67. Jyothirmayi GN, Reddi AS. Effect of diltiazem on glomerular heparan sulfate and albuminuria in diabetic rats. *Hypertension* 1993; 21(6 Part I):765–802.

68. Munter K, Kirchengast M. Individual and combined effects of verapamil or trandolopril on glomeruloprotection in the stroke prone rat. *J Am Soc Nephrol* 1996; 7:681–686.

69. Bakris GL, Mangrum A, Copley JB, Vicknair N. Calcium channel or beta blockade on progression of diabetic renal disease in African Americans. *Hypertension* 1997:(in press).

70. Gilbert RE, Jerums G, Allen T, et al. Effect of different antihypertensive agents on normotensive microalbuminuric patients with IDDM and NIDDM [abstract]. *J Am Soc Nephrol* 1994; 5:377.

71. Hartmann A, Lund K, Hagel L, et al. Contrasting short-term effects of nifedipine on glomerular and tubular functions in glomerulonephritic patietns. *J Am Soc Nephrol* 1994; 5:1385–1391.

72. Velussi M, Brocco E, Frigato F, et al. Effects of cilazapril and amlodipine on kidney function in hypertensive NIDDM patients. *Diabetes* 1996; 45:216–222.

73. Veniant M, Heudes D, Clozel JP, et al. Calcium blockade versus ACE inhibition in clipped and unclipped kidneys of 2K-1C rats. *Kidney Int* 1994; 46:421–429.

74. Wenzel RO, Helmchen U, Schoeppe W, Schwietzer G. Combination treatment of enalapril with nitrendipine in rats with renovascular hypertension. *Hypertension* 1994; 23:114–122.

75. Bakris GL. Effects of diltiazem or lisinopril on massive proteinuria associated with diabetes mellitus. *Ann Intern Med* 1990; 112(9):707–708.

76. Epstein M, Bakris GL. Newer approaches to antihypertensive therapy using fixed dose combination therapy: future perspectives. *Arch Intern Med* 1996; 156:1969–1978.

77. Morgan TO, Anderson A. Hemodynamic comparison on enalapril and felodipine and their combination. *Kidney Int* 1992; 36:S78–S81.

78. Salvetti A, Innocenti PF, Iardella M, et al. Captopril and nifedipine interactions in the treatment of essential hypertensives: a crossover study. *J Hypertens Suppl* 1987; 5(4):S139–S142.

79. Bakris GL, Barnhill BW, Sadler R. Treatment of arterial hypertension in diabetic humans: importance of therapeutic selection. *Kidney Int* 1992; 41(4):912–919.

80. Bakris GL. Renal effects of calcium antagonists in diabetes mellitus: an overview of studies in animal models and in humans. *Am J Hypertens* 1991; 4(Suppl II):487S–493S.

81. National Hight Blood Pressure Education Program Working Group on Hypertension and Renal Disease. 1995 update of the working group reports on chronic renal failure and renovascular hypertension. *Arch Intern Med* 1996; 156:1938–1947.

CHAPTER 13

Combination Therapy for Stroke: Lessons from STOP-Hypertension

Lennart Hansson

Arterial hypertension increases the risk of cardiovascular, cerebral, and renal morbidity (1). By lowering elevated arterial pressure, stroke, and, to a lesser degree, coronary heart disease, morbidity and mortality are positively affected (2). It may appear that these beneficial effects have been obtained mainly with diuretics and β-adrenoceptor blocking agents, as shown in a meta-analysis of 13 large prospective intervention trials in hypertension (2).

However, the real breakthrough with regard to demonstrating benefits of pharmacological antihypertensive treatment was the results obtained with treating patients with malignant hypertension (3). Many of these studies in the 1950s and early 1960s were conducted—and some were even published—before diuretics became clinically available in 1958 (4), and certainly a decade or more before the first reports of the antihypertensive effect of β-blockers were published in 1964 (5, 6).

It is true, though, that evidence is still lacking that the newer classes of antihypertensive agents (i.e., the ACE inhibitors and the calcium antagonists) reduce cardiovascular morbidity and mortality. Prospective intervention trials with such agents are currently in progress (7–11) and some of these will be briefly discussed here. Three recently published case-control studies (12–14) dealing with comparisons of various antihypertensive drug classes regarding their effect on coronary heart disease (CHD) morbidity are of some interest in this context, partly because they neglect to bring up the effect of antihypertensive treatment on stroke morbidity.

When evaluating the available data from prospective, randomized intervention trials in hypertension, the following conclusions can be made:

1. The reduction in blood pressure per se is associated with reductions in cardiovascular morbidity and mortality.
2. The preventive effect of antihypertensive treatment against stroke has always been more impressive than the effect against CHD.

3. The positive results in this regard have, almost without exception, been obtained with combinations of antihypertensive drugs.
4. In elderly hypertensives, the effect of antihypertensive treatment assumes particular importance since stroke morbidity and mortality are relatively more common than in young and middle-age hypertensives.

The positive findings in the Swedish Trial in Old Patients with Hypertension (STOP-Hypertension) (15) of combined antihypertensive treatment on stroke morbidity and mortality will be discussed in somewhat greater detail here.

STOP-Hypertension

STOP-Hypertension was a double-blind, placebo-controlled trial of antihypertensive therapy in "old/elderly" hypertensive patients (i.e., men and women age 70 to 84 years). The main results have been published in detail before (15). In brief, antihypertensive treatment based on one of three β-blockers (atenolol, metoprolol, or pindolol) and/or a diuretic combination (hydrochlorothiazide and amiloride) caused highly significant reductions in all primary endpoints, stroke, and total mortality (Table 13-1) (15).

It should be noted that most patients (66%) were taking combined therapy of one of the β-blockers and the diuretic combination. No attempt has been made to analyze possible differences in outcome between the four therapeutic alternatives, since patients were not randomized to one of these. Randomization was only between active treatment and placebo.

THE STROKE-PREVENTIVE EFFECT

The annual incidence of stroke in the STOP-Hypertension study was estimated by using a Poisson model (16) taking current age, gender, treatment, systolic blood pressure, and diastolic blood pressure into account for all patients in the study. The constants of the model were estimated by the maximum likelihood method. The risk of stroke was found to be significantly lower for a patient on active antihypertensive

TABLE 13-1. MAIN RESULTS OF STOP-HYPERTENSION

Results	Percent Reduction	p-value
Deaths, all causes	43	.0079
Stroke, all	47	.0081
CHD	13 (myocardial infarction)	ns
CV events, all*	40	.0031

CHD = coronary heart disease; CV-cardiovascular; ns=not significant.
*Fatal and nonfatal strokes, myocardial infarcts, and other cardiovascular mortalities.
(Adapted from Dahlöf and colleagues [15], with permission.)

treatment than for a patient on placebo having the same in-study blood pressure, age, and gender (42%, p = .0402) (17).

The annual incidence of stroke for a man age 75 with a systolic blood pressure of 175 mmHg on placebo or active combined antihypertensive therapy over a range of diastolic blood pressures (70 to 100 mmHg) is illustrated in Figure 13-1. The corresponding data for women are shown in Figure 13-2.

The explanation for this additional benefit of antihypertensive treatment (i.e., a preventive effect against stroke over and above the effect obtained by lowering the blood pressure) is not immediately apparent. In the original report the possible importance of using a combined antihypertensive therapeutic regimen (β-blocker and potassium-sparing diuretic combination) was brought up (17). Other investigators have later discussed the potential benefits of antihypertensive treatment with potassium-sparing diuretics for the prevention of sudden cardiac death (14, 18). In the STOP-Hypertension study, a numerically lower but statistically insignificant rate of cardiac events was found in men and women on active antihypertensive treatment as compared to placebo for the same blood pressure and age (17), which would tend to support the importance of sparing potassium in terms of preventing cardiac events, possibly by reducing the risk of arrhythmias. However, there is no obvious mechanism for a preventive effect against stroke that is related to potassium sparing. In animal experiments, Tobian and associates (19) have reported a protective effect of potassium against vascular complications that is unrelated to the level of blood pressure. The underlying mechanism of this positive effect remains to be elucidated, though.

Some support for these findings (i.e., a lower rate of stroke in treated patients for the same level of blood pressure) can be found in a subgroup analysis of the European Working Party against High Blood Pressure in the Elderly (EWPHE) study (20), No mechanism to explain this finding was suggested. It should also be mentioned that, in contrast to the findings in the STOP-Hypertension study (17) and in the EWPHE study (20), however, the Australian National Blood Pressure study in mild hypertension found that the rate of cardiovascular complications in the actively treated patients did not quite fall to the level seen in patients on placebo with the same blood pressures (21).

CONCLUSIONS

In the STOP-Hypertension study, a marked reduction in fatal and nonfatal stroke (47%) was seen in the actively treated group. The risk of stroke was significantly lower in actively treated patients than in those taking placebo (42%), even for the same level of blood pressure. There is some support for this finding in the EWPHE study, but the mechanism for this beneficial effect is not clear. It is conceivable that the antihypertensive therapy used in the STOP-Hypertension study (i.e., a combination of β-blockade and a thiazide with a po-

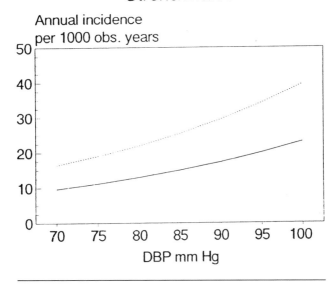

Figure 13-1. *Annual incidence of stroke per 1,000 observation-years in the STOP-Hypertension study for men age 75 years with a systolic blood pressure of 175 mmHg. Placebo (dotted line); active treatment (solid line). (From Ekbom and colleagues [17], with permission.)*

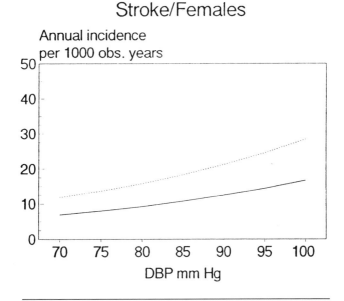

Figure 13-2. *Annual incidence of stroke per 1,000 observation-years in the STOP-Hypertension Study for women age 75 years with a systolic blood pressure of 175 mmHg. Placebo (dotted line); active treatment (solid line). (From Ekbom and colleagues [17], with permission.)*

tassium-sparing component) may be of relevance in this context, but this remains to be fully elucidated. From a practical and clinical point of view, though, the stroke-preventive effect of a combined antihypertensive regime, such as the one used in the STOP-Hypertension study, has been proven beyond doubt.

REFERENCES

1. Stokes III J, Kannel WB, Wolf PA, et al. The relative importance of selected risk factors for various manifestations of cardiovascular disease among men and women from 35 to 64 years old: 30 years of follow-up in the Framingham study. *Circulation* 1987; 75(Suppl V):65–73.

2. Collins R, Peto R, MacMahon S, et al. Blood pressure, stroke, and coronary heart disease. Part 2, short-term reductions in blood pressure: overview of randomised drug trials in their epidemiological context. *Lancet* 1990; 335:827–838.

3. Hansson L. The J-shaped curve and how far should blood pressure be lowered? In: Laragh JH, Brenner BM, eds. *Hypertension: pathophysiology, diagnosis and management.* 2nd ed. New York: Raven Press, 1995: 2765–2770.

4. Beyer KH. The mechanism of action of chlorothiazide. *Ann N Y Acad Sci* 1958; 71:363–371.

5. Prichard BNC. Hypotensive action of pronethalol. *Br Med J* 1964; I:1227.

6. Prichard BNC, Gillam PMS. Use of propranolol ("inderal") in treatment of hypertension. *Br Med J* 1964; II:725–727.

7. Dahlöf B, Hansson L, Lindholm LH, et al. STOP-Hypertension-2: a prospective intervention trial of "newer" versus "older" treatment alternatives in old patients with hypertension. *Blood Press* 1993; 2:136–141.

8. The CAPPP Group. The captopril prevention project: a prospective intervention trial of angiotensin converting enzyme inhibition in the treatment of hypertension. *J Hypertension* 1990; 8:985–990.

9. The NORDIL Study Group. The nordic diltiazem study. An intervention study in hypertension comparing calcium antagonist based treatment with conventional therapy. *Blood Press* 1993; 2:312–321.

10. Amery A, Birkenhäger W, Bulpitt CJ, et al. SYST-EUR. A multicentre trial on the treatment of isolated systolic hypertension in the elderly: objectives, protocol, and organisation. *Aging* 1991; 3:287–302.

11. Cushman WC for the ALLHAT Research Group. The antihypertensive and lipid lowering treatment to prevent heart attack trial (ALLHAT)—design and initial characteristics [abstract]. *Hypertension* 1995; 25:4.

12. Psaty BM, Heckbert SR, Koepsell TD, et al. The risk of myocardial infarction associated with antihypertensive drug therapies. *JAMA* 1995; 274:620–625.

13. Aursnes I, Litleskare I, Frøyland H, Abdelnoor M. Association between various drugs used for hypertension and risk of acute myocardial infarction. *Blood Press* 1995; 4:157–163.

14. Hoes AW, Grobbee DE, Lubsen J, et al. Diuretics, β-blockers, and the risk of sudden death in hypertensive patients. *Ann Intern Med* 1995; 123:481–487.

15. Dahlöf B, Lindholm LH, Hansson L, et al. Morbidity and mortality in the Swedish Trial in Old Patients with Hypertension (STOP-hypertension). *Lancet* 1991; 338: 1281–1285.

16. Breslow NE, Day NE. *Statistical methods in cancer research*. Vol. II. No. 32. Lyon: IARC Scientific Publications, 1987: 131–135.

17. Ekbom T, Dahlöf B, Hansson L, et al. The stroke preventive effect in elderly hypertensives cannot be fully explained by the reduction in office blood pressure—insights from the Swedish Trial in Old Patients with Hypertension (STOP-Hypertension). *Blood Press* 1992; 1:168–172.

18. Siscovick DS, Raghunathan TE, Psaty BM, et al. Diuretic therapy for hypertension and the risk of primary cardiac arrest. *N Engl J Med* 1994; 330:1852–1857.

19. Tobian L, Sugimoto T, Johnson MA. High K diets protect against endothelial injury in stroke prone SHR rats. *J Hypertens* 1987; 5(Suppl 5):263–265.

20. Staessen J, Bulpitt C, Clement D, et al. Relation between mortality and treated blood pressure in the elderly patients with hypertension: report of the European Working Party on High Blood Pressure in the Elderly. *Br Med J* 1989; 298:1552–1556.

21. Australian Therapeutic Trial in Mild Hypertension Management Committee. The Australian therapeutic trial in mild hypertension. *Lancet* 1980; i;1261–1267.

CHAPTER 14

Combination Therapy: Impact on Cardiovascular Disease Risk Factors

Myron H. Weinberger

The reduction of blood pressure has been shown, unequivocally, to reduce the overall occurrence of cardiovascular complications related to hypertension. However a raging debate has been in progress for two decades regarding the impact of specific antihypertensive therapy on different cardiovascular events and the possibility of variable benefit from individual antihypertensive drugs at the same level of blood pressure reduction. This debate continues today and is being tested by a variety of ongoing studies. It is not the purpose of this chapter to review the existing evidence or to describe the myriad issues and studies involved. Rather, this chapter will examine the risk factor surrogates for many of these forms of cardiovascular disease and the current knowledge regarding the impact of specific drug categories and their combinations on these risk factors. Presumably the risk factor alterations may enable the prediction of subsequent cardiovascular event outcomes, a concept that may be validated by the future results of studies now in progress.

The risk factors that this chapter will consider include blood pressure itself, the lipoprotein profile, insulin sensitivity and carbohydrate tolerance, uric acid levels, renal function, LVH—all independent risk factors for cardiovascular disease that have been shown to be influenced by specific antihypertensive agents. In addition, the effect of single and combination drug therapy on the electrolytes that have been implicated in cardiac arrhythmias, potassium and magnesium, will also be discussed. While extensive evidence regarding the impact of these agents as monotherapy on these risk factors is available, less information has been obtained for combination therapy. Thus in many instances extrapolation may be required to estimate the effect of certain drug combinations on these risk factors. The presentation will be organized by initially describing the effect of single-drug treatment, separated into the following therapeutic categories of agents most commonly used at present: diuretics, antisympathetic agents (central alpha-adrenergic agonists, ganglionic blocking agents, peripheral alpha-adrenergic blockers and beta-adrenergic blocking drugs) and vasodilators (direct-acting agents, ACE inhibitors, angiotensin II receptor antagonists, and calcium channel entry blocking agents). Then the evidence for the effect of specific combination drug therapy will be presented and, for combinations for which data are unavailable, discussion of the likely impact will be provided.

BLOOD PRESSURE

While the goal of antihypertensive therapy is obviously to reduce blood pressure, all antihypertensive agents are not equal in their efficacy (1). An extensive bibliography attests to differences in blood pressure response rates to different drugs, in general, and to heterogeneity of response to these agents on the basis of a variety of demographic, environmental, and physiological factors. As a general rule, the response rates of monotherapeutic agents in an unselected population of hypertensive patients seldom exceeds 60%, and for several agents response rates substantially lower than 50% are commonly observed (1). One exception to this is the consistently high (>70%) response rate to calcium channel entry blockers when used in adequate doses (2). In some studies the response rates to usual doses of agents given alone can be increased by increasing the dose to maximal levels, often associated with an increased likelihood of side effects. For this reason, many experts favor combination therapy to achieve effective blood pressure control with less-than-maximal doses of the two drugs chosen, thus likely to reduce the occurrence of side effects.

Because of the differences in mechanisms of action of various antihypertensive agents and of the heterogeneity in response to these drugs, not all combinations have equivalent blood pressure-lowering efficacy. In general, combining diuretics with other classes of antihypertensives provides enhanced blood pressure reduction in comparison to monotherapy with either agent. One exception to this observation is the combination of calcium channel entry blocker and diuretic, which has been found by most investigators not to have additive effects when the calcium channel blocker is given first (3). In general, combining two drugs of the antisympathetic group, with the exception of peripheral alpha- and beta-adrenergic receptor blockers, has minimal additive effects. In contrast, the combination of two agents from the vasodilator class is typically quite effective, particularly when ACE inhibitors are combined with calcium channel entry blockers. The use of the direct-acting agents, hydralazine (Apresoline) and minoxidil (Loniten), is generally reserved for "third-step" therapy because of the multitude of side effects associated with these agents and the need for treatment of the tachycardia resulting from sympathetic stimulation, and the volume expansion and fluid retention invariably accompanying these potent drugs.

LIPIDS AND LIPOPROTEINS

Emerging data from a variety of epidemiological and interventional studies indicate that lipid and lipoprotein levels are major determinants of cardiovascular disease (4–7). Not only are these components major factors in the pathogenesis of coronary artery disease, angina, and myocardial infarction, but they also have been linked to stroke and renal disease. The initial lipid abnormality identified as an independent risk factor for heart disease was the total cholesterol level. Recent evidence from the Multiple Risk Factor Intervention Trial screening data indicates an increased risk for cardiovascular mortality at levels of total cholesterol above 180 mg/dl in men (6). In addition to total cholesterol, the high-density lipoprotein (HDL) component has been shown to have even greater predictive value, with low levels (≤40 mg/dl in men) being associated with an increased risk for heart attack (7). This has led to the use of a ratio of total cholesterol to HDL as a way of assessing risk more precisely. Additional lipid risk factors have emerged in more recent studies, including triglycerides and lipoprotein (a). The risk of the commonly measured lipids, total cholesterol, HDL, and triglycerides can be assessed by the derived measurement of low-density lipoprotein (LDL), which is calculated from the other three measurements.

While the evidence for these components as risk factors for cardiovascular disease has come primarily from epidemiological observations, more recent intervention trials have confirmed their importance. It has been consistently shown that lowering of total cholesterol and LDL is associated with a decreased risk of myocardial infarction as a primary event in high-risk individuals and in recurrence of disease in secondary prevention trials. At present the link between lipids and stroke or renal disease is based primarily on observational data and has not been confirmed by interventional trials, by and large.

The effects of antihypertensive drugs on the lipid profile is summarized in Table 14-1. In general, all diuretics raise total cholesterol and triglycerides in a dose-dependent fashion (8). Despite frequent misconceptions, loop diuretics, such as furosemide, have these adverse lipid effects when they are administered three or more times a day, as is required for antihypertensive efficacy. There is some evidence that newer diuretics such as indapamide and torasemide may not produce adverse lipid effects at doses that do lower blood pressure when given as monotherapy (9). However, for the most commonly used diuretic, hydrochlorothiazide, the antihypertensive effect requires a dose of 25 mg/d or more (when used alone) and lipid changes are seen at that level. Some have argued that the adverse lipid effects of diuretics are transient, a view not supported by most parallel, placebo-controlled trials or by observations made following discontinuation of diuretic therapy. In order to avoid the lipid-raising effect of diuretics, it is often necessary to lower the dose to a level that does not effectively control blood pressure. Thus low-dose diuretic therapy is usually combined with other antihypertensive agents, as will be discussed.

TABLE 14-1. THE EFFECTS OF ANTIHYPERTENSIVE AGENTS ON LIPIDS

Antihypertensive Agent	TC	TG	HDL
Diuretics (dose dependent)	↑3 to 11%	↑10 to 20%	NC
Central alpha agonists	NC	?	NC
Ganglionic blockers	?	?	?
Peripheral alpha antagonists	↓4%	↓8%	↑4%
Beta-blockers	↑0 to 5%	↑8 to 25%	↓5 to 20%
with ISA pindolol	NC	↓10%	↑10%
ACE inhibitors	NC	NC	NC
Angiotensin II receptor blockers	NC	NC	NC
Calcium channel entry blockers	NC	NC	NC
Hydralazine, minoxidil	(rarely given alone; effects ?)		

↑ = increase; ↓ = decrease; NC = no change; ? = uncertain; ISA = intrinsic sympathomimetic activity; TC = total cholesterol; TG = triglyceride ; HDL = high-density lipoprotein component.
(Modified from Opie, Frishman. *Drugs for the heart.* 4th ed. Philadelphia: Saunders, 1995: p. 292.)

In general, the centrally acting alpha-adrenergic agonists have no consistent effects on total cholesterol or HDL and insufficient evidence regarding their effect on triglycerides is available (8). Very little is known concerning the lipid effects of ganglionic blocking agents, drugs that are rarely used as monotherapy because of their side effects. On the other hand, most beta-adrenergic blocking agents, with the exception of those having intrinsic sympathomimetic activity (ISA), have a profound effect on lipids, modestly elevating total cholesterol and especially triglycerides and, perhaps most importantly, lowering HDL levels (8, 10). These effects are seen regardless of cardioselective or nonselective blockade. This implies that either the beta receptor has a favorable lipid action or that sympathetic stimulation of the alpha receptor, which is unopposed when beta blockers are given, has an adverse effect. Evidence in support of the latter concept can be seen by examining the effect of peripheral alpha-adrenergic receptor blockade, which produces lipid effects exactly opposite those of beta-blockers (8, 11). The alpha-blockers consistently lower total cholesterol and triglycerides, and are among the few agents that have been shown to raise HDL. In general, the ACE inhibitors, angiotensin II receptor blockers, and calcium channel entry blockers have not been shown to have either beneficial or adverse effects on lipids when given alone. Less information is available regarding the direct-acting vasodilators, hydralazine and minoxidil, since these agents are almost invariably combined with diuretics to combat fluid retention, and beta-blockers to reduce the tachycardia resulting from sympathetic stimulation. One could presume that, because of the marked sympathetic stimulation resulting from the administration of hydralazine or minoxidil, these agents would have an adverse effect on lipids by themselves.

When diuretics are combined with beta-blockers, the adverse effects of the diuretic on total cholesterol and triglycerides is accentuated and compounded by the effect of beta-blockers to lower HDL. The combination of bisoprolol and hydrochlorothiazide (Ziac) may be a notable exception to this statement, perhaps owing to the low doses of each agent used in the combined preparation. The adverse lipid effects of diuretic therapy are blunted or prevented when the drugs are combined with either peripheral alpha-adrenergic blocking agents or ACE inhibitors (12, 13). The metabolic effects of combined diuretic and angiotensin II receptor blocker therapy have not been extensively evaluated. As might be predicted from the previous discussion regarding the lipid effects of alpha- and beta-blockers when used as monotherapy, when they are combined (alpha- and beta-blockers such as labetalol) the lipid effects tend to be neither beneficial nor adverse (8).

INSULIN SENSITIVITY AND CARBOHYDRATE TOLERANCE

Diabetes has long been known to be an independent risk factor for cardiovascular disease (14). More recently less-severe abnormalities of carbohydrate tolerance have been identified and linked to insulin resistance and hypertension (15). It appears that a substantial number of hypertensive subjects have absolute or relative insulin resistance and thus are likely to have subtle abnormalities of carbohydrate metabolism and to be susceptible to the development of overt type II NIDDM. This susceptibility may be modulated by the effects of antihypertensive drug therapy, several agents of which are known to influence insulin sensitivity and carbohydrate tolerance (9, 11). Diuretics may worsen insulin sensitivity in a variety of ways, including alterations in insulin release, reducing insulin's action by electrolyte depletion or hemodynamic factors, or perhaps by a direct action of the agents on glucose-insulin dynamics (9). In some but not all studies of the effects of diuretics on carbohydrate tolerance, the adverse effects can be attenuated by the use of potassium supplementation or potassium-sparing diuretic formulations (16). As is true for many of the other metabolic effects of diuretic therapy, the manifestations on carbohydrate sensitivity are dose dependent and appear to be less severe with agents such as indapamide and torasemide (9).

Beta-adrenergic blocking drugs also worsen insulin sensitivity, although the mechanism for this effect is not clearly understood. It has been suggested that insulin release from the beta cells of the pancreas is mediated by beta-adrenergic stimulation. In addition, a hemodynamic effect induced by the vasoconstriction that occurs with beta-blockade in the vasculature of skeletal muscle may also be operative (17). This hypothesis is consistent with observations with the use of alpha-adrenergic blocking drugs, which have been shown to improve insulin sensitivity and carbohydrate tolerance (18). These agents act to dilate the resistance vessels in the skeletal muscle bed and thus provide greater surface area for the action of insulin to promote glucose uptake. This beneficial effect of alpha-blockade on insulin sensitivity is readily observed by the improvement in carbohydrate tolerance as well as blood pressure reduction in diabetic hypertensives treated with alpha-blockers (18). ACE inhibitors have also been shown to improve insulin sensitivity and carbohydrate tolerance, presumably by a hemodynamic effect involving vasodilation and increased blood flow to the muscle bed (13). Less information is available concerning the effects of the new angiotensin II receptor blockers. Calcium channel blockers probably have no distinct or consistent effect on insulin sensitivity or carbohydrate tolerance, although limited information suggests that insulin secretion can be inhibited by these agents in experimental settings. On the other hand, at least one study has found an improvement in insulin sensitivity in insulin-resistant subjects after receiving the dihydropyridine calcium channel blocker amlodipine (19).

The effects of combination antihypertensive therapy on insulin sensitivity and carbohydrate tolerance have not been carefully evaluated. Since both diuretics and beta-blockers have adverse effects on insulin sensitivity that appear to be mediated, at least in part, by different mechanisms, it would seem logical that there would be an additive adverse effect of the combination. On the other hand, limited observations indicate that the combination of diuretic and alpha-blocker or diuretic and ACE inhibitor tend to be associated with an attenuation of the adverse effects of the diuretic alone on carbohydrate tolerance (13).

URIC ACID

Some recent epidemiological evidence has implicated uric acid as an individual risk factor for cardiovascular disease (20, 21). Extensive confirmation of these reports is not yet available nor is there any evidence from interventional studies to confirm a causal role. Finally, a clear pathophysiological role is also lacking, making it more likely that uric acid elevations may be a marker for another factor. Nevertheless, some antihypertensive agents are known to influence uric acid metabolism and thus this factor is deserving of comment. Diuretics have long been known to increase uric acid levels in blood and to provoke gouty attacks in susceptible individuals (22). This effect appears to be a generic one which is dose dependent. Thus even furosemide, when given with the frequency required to lower blood pressure, is capable of raising blood levels. There is some evidence that low doses of indapamide and torasemide have minimal effects on uric acid. Two groups of drugs have been reported to have a uricosuric action: ACE inhibitors and angiotensin II receptor blockers (23, 24). These observations implicate a renal tubular effect of angiotensin II in uric acid reabsorption. The effects of these agents appear to be more marked in the presence of elevated blood uric acid levels (23). Combining ACE inhibitors with diuretics attenuates the diuretic-associated increase in uric acid (13), and presumably the combination of angiotensin II receptor blocker and diuretic should have a similar effect.

RENAL FUNCTION

Untreated hypertension is associated with the development and progression of renal disease. It has long been assumed that blood pressure reduction with antihypertensive therapy should reduce the risk of renal disease and/or halt its progression. A substantial body of evidence suggests that this is not invariably the case. Several studies document progression of renal disease to end-stage renal failure despite apparent adequate blood pressure control (25). Studies are currently in progress to discern whether this observation can be explained on the basis of racial factors, level of blood pressure control, or the specific form of antihypertensive therapy utilized. Since renal function is influenced by systemic and renal blood pressure, renal blood flow, vasoconstrictor and vasodilatory factors, extracellular fluid volume, and, perhaps, circulating lipid levels, it is probable that the impact of specific antihypertensive therapy on the kidney is complex. Diuretics may reduce renal function in the setting of contraction of extracellular fluid volume and reduced glomerular filtration rate. Moreover, these agents stimulate the renin-angiotensin and sympathetic nervous systems, further reducing glomerular filtration. Associated elevation of lipids with diuretic therapy could further reduce renal function in susceptible individuals. Beta-adrenergic blocking agents have been shown to reduce renal function, presumably as a result of an increase in renal vascular resistance (26). On the other hand, agents that decrease renal vascular resistance, such as alpha-adrenergic blocking drugs, ACE inhibitors, calcium channel entry blockers, and, presumably, angiotensin II receptor blockers, appear to improve renal function and could potentially reduce the likelihood of developing renal disease.

While the ACE inhibitors have been shown to be effective in delaying the progression of diabetic renal disease in those with mild renal impairment or microalbuminuria (27), it is unlikely that this group of drugs will be the only one found to have such beneficial effects on renal function. A variety of studies utilizing calcium channel entry blockers suggest that some of these agents as well can reduce diabetic renal disease progression (28). It is likely that similar observations will be reported in the future with the angiotensin II receptor blockers.

LEFT VENTRICULAR HYPERTROPHY

Left ventricular hypertrophy has been shown to be a risk factor for cardiovascular disease in many epidemiological studies (29). The mechanisms proposed to explain this relationship include an increased risk of coronary ischemia and myocardial infarction resulting from a supply-demand mismatch induced by the increased myocardial mass, progression of hemodynamic compromise to congestive heart failure, and the increased susceptibility to cardiac arrhythmias engendered by the enlarged ventricle (30). Less information is at hand regarding the beneficial effects of inducing regression of LVH (31). Since hypertension is the major contributing factor for cardiac hypertrophy, it has long been assumed that blood pressure reduction per se would suffice to reduce hypertension-related LVH. Analyses of recent studies would suggest that this is not necessarily a valid assumption and that the drugs used to lower blood pressure may have variable effects on the regression of LVH (32). In view of new information identifying not only pressure as a factor in the pathogenesis of LVH, but also sodium balance, extracellular fluid volume, and, more importantly, the activity of components of the renin-angiotensin-aldosterone and sympathetic nervous systems, it is not surprising that not all antihypertensive agents have equal efficacy in the reduction of cardiac hypertrophy (32, 33).

Recent meta-analyses have suggested hierarchial effects of different classes of antihypertensive agents on regression of hypertensive LVH, with diuretics having a relatively weak effect, followed by central sympathetic agonists, beta-blockers, alpha-blockers, calcium channel entry blockers, and ACE inhibitors used as monotherapy (32). The role of angiotensin II receptor blockers is not yet clear. Thus most studies suggest that the greatest and most consistent demonstration of regression of LVH can be seen with calcium channel entry blockers and ACE inhibitors alone. It would be anticipated that when these agents are used in combination, even greater reductions in left ventricular mass may be seen. This has not yet been clearly identified however. Similarly, intuitive reasoning would lead one to predict that virtually all combinations of these classes of antihypertensive agents should have additive effects on the regression of LVH, but this has not been clearly demonstrated. Suffice it to say that there is no convincing evidence in humans that combination antihypertensive therapy can worsen LVH. From experimental studies in animals it is conceivable that combinations of diuretics and direct-acting vasodilators (hydralazine, minoxidil) could exacerbate LVH because of the ability of both agents to markedly stimulate the renin-angiotensin-aldosterone and sympathetic nervous systems in the absence of pharmacologic restraint (34).

ELECTROLYTES: POTASSIUM AND MAGNESIUM

Diuretics have long been known to induce potassium and magnesium wasting (20). These effects are dose dependent and are linked to the level of sodium intake, the degree of activation of the renin-angiotensin-aldosterone system, and to renal function. While the role of diuretic-induced hypokalemia and hypomagnesemia in inducing cardiac arrhythmias has been a subject of vigorous debate and controversy, recent observations suggest that diuretics lacking potassium- and magnesium-sparing characteristics are associated with an increased risk of sudden death (35, 36). Studies of potassium supplementation have been less convincing, perhaps owing to failure to replete intracellular potassium stores, which generally requires magnesium repletion to accomplish. Beta-adrenergic blocking agents can increase serum potassium concentration, but usually only to a minimal degree (0.2 to 0.4 mmol/L). ACE inhibitors have been shown to increase serum potassium concentration, presumably by inhibiting aldosterone production only in subjects with renal impairment or in those with hypoaldosteronism, such as is seen in the elderly or in association with diabetic renal disease. Although there is limited data at present, it is reasonable to assume that angiotensin II receptor blockers would have similar effects. The other antihypertensive classes, in general, have no consistent effects on potassium or magnesium metabolism. While the calcium channel entry blockers do not influence potassium or magnesium metabolism, agents such as verapamil and diltiazem, but not the dihydropyridine agents, are known to have an antiarrhythmic effect in the presence of supraventricular arrhythmias. In addition, the sympathetic stimulation induced by hydralazine and minoxidil could be expected to stimulate arrhythmogenesis, particularly in susceptible individuals.

The dependence of diuretic-induced potassium loss on the activity of the renin-aldosterone system can be documented from the observation that combining diuretics and ACE inhibitors prevents diuretic-induced hypokalemia (13). Moreover, this mechanism for preservation of potassium stores when this combination is used may contribute to the beneficial effects of the combination on carbohydrate tolerance, as described earlier.

SUMMARY AND CONCLUSIONS

When blood pressure control is not achieved with a modest dose of a single antihypertensive agent, it is often preferable to add a second drug rather than to increase the dose of the initial agent to its maximum, since fewer dose-dependent side effects are likely to occur. The choice of an antihypertensive drug combination is guided by likely efficacy as well as the impact of the agents used on other cardiovascular disease risk factors that may be present or be matters of concern. In general, one can anticipate an additive antihypertensive effect when diuretics are combined with most other types of antihypertensive agents, with the possible exception of calcium channel entry blockers. However, when one wishes to minimize the effects of antihypertensive therapy on the lipid profile, insulin sensitivity and carbohydrate tolerance, uric acid levels, renal function, LVH and electrolyte metabolism, it appears that the combination of ACE inhibitor with either a diuretic or a calcium channel entry blocker would be most desirable. It is likely that similar beneficial impact will be observed by combining the new angiotensin II receptor blockers with diuretics and perhaps other agents as well, but the documentation of their interactive effects remains to be reported.

REFERENCES

1. Chobanian AV. Antihypertensive therapy in evolution. *N Engl J Med* 1986; 314:1701–1702.

2. Weinberger MH. The case for calcium-channel blockers in hypertension. *Int Med* 1993; 17:9–16.

3. Weinberger MH. Additive effects of diuretics or sodium restriction with calcium channel blockers in the treatment of hypertension. *J Cardiovasc Pharmacol* 1988; 12(Suppl 4):S72–S75.

4. Castelli WP. Epidemiology of coronary heart disease: the Framingham study. *Am J Med* 1984; 76(Suppl 2A):4-12.

5. Lipid Research Clinics Program. The Lipid Research Clinics Coronary Primary Prevention Trial results: reduction in incidence of coronary heart disease. *JAMA* 1984; 251:351–364.

6. Multiple Risk Factor Intervention Trial Research Group. Multiple Risk Factor Intervention Trial: risk factor changes and mortality results. *JAMA* 1982;248:1465–1477.

7. Gordon T, Castelli WP, Hjortland MC, et al. High-density lipoprotein as a protective factor against coronary heart disease: the Framingham study. *Am J Med* 1977; 62:707–714.

8. Weinberger MH. Antihypertensive therapy and lipids: evidence, mechanisms and implications. *Arch Intern Med* 1985; 145:1102–1105.

9. Weinberger MH. Mechanisms of diuretic effects on carbohydrate tolerance, insulin sensitivity and lipid levels. *Eur Heart J* 1992; 13(Suppl G):5–9.

10. Weinberger MH. Potential benefit of combination therapy with diuretics and beta blockers having intrinsic sympathomimetic activity. *Eur Heart J* 1990; 11:560–565.

11. Weinberger MH. Antihypertensive therapy and lipids: paradoxical influences on cardiovascular disease risk. *Am J Med* 1986; 80(Suppl 2A):64–70.

12. Johnson BF, Romero L, Johnson J. Comparative effects of propranolol and prazosin upon serum lipids in thiazide-treated hypertensive patients. *Am J Med* 1984; 76:109–114.

13. Weinberger MH. Comparison of captopril and hydrochlorothiazide alone and in combination in mild-to-moderate essential hypertension. *Br J Clin Pharmacol* 1982; 14:127s–131s.

14. Kannel WB, McGee DL. Diabetes and cardiovascular risk factors: the Framingham study. *Circulation* 1979; 59:8–13.

15. Modan M, Halkin H, Almog S, et al. Hyperinsulinemia: a link between hypertension, obesity, and glucose intolerance. *J Clin Invest* 1985; 75:809–817.

16. Helderman JH, Elahi D, Andersen DK. Prevention of the glucose intolerance of thiazide diuretics by maintenance of body potassium. *Diabetes* 1983; 32:106–111.

17. Laakso M, Edelman SV, Brechtel G, Baron AD. Decreased effect of insulin to stimulate skeletal muscle blood flow in obese man: a novel mechanism for insulin resistance. *J Clin Invest* 1990; 85:1844–1852.

18. Dominguez LJ, Weinberger MH, Cefalu WT, et al. Doxazosin improves insulin sensitivity and lowers blood pressure in type II diabetic hypertensives with no changes in tyrosine kinase activity or insulin binding. *Am J Hypertens* 1995; 8:528–532.

19. Beer NA, Jakubowicz DJ, Beer RM, Nestler JE. The calcium channel blocker amlodipine raises serum dehydroepiandrosterone

sulfate and androstenedione but lowers serum cortisol, in insulin-resistant obese and hypertensive men. *J Clin Endocrinol Metab* 1993; 76:1464–1469.

20. Persky VW, Dyer AR, Idris-Stoven E, et al. Uric acid: a risk factor for coronary heart disease? *Circulation* 1979; 59:969–977.

21. Brand FN, McGee DL, Kannel WB, et al. Hyperuricemia as a risk factor of coronary heart disease: the Framingham study. *Am J Epidemiol* 1985; 121:11–18.

22. Weinberger MH. Diuretics and their side effects: dilemma in the treatment of hypertension. *Hypertension* 1988; 11(Suppl II):II-16–II-20.

23. Leary WP, Reyes AJ, Acosta-Barrios TN, Maharaj B. Captopril once daily as monotherapy in patients with hyperuricaemia and essential hypertension. *Lancet* 1985; i:277–281.

24. Nakashima M, Uematsu T, Kosuge K, Kanam M. Pilot study of the uricosuric effect of Dup-753, a new angiotensin II receptor antagonist, in healthy subjects. *Eur J Clin Pharmacol* 1992; 42:333–335.

25. Rostand SG, Kirk KA, Rutsky EA. Racial differences in the incidence of treatment for end-stage renal disease. *N Engl J Med* 1982; 306:1276–1289.

26. Bauer JH, Brooks CS. The long-term effect of propranolol therapy on renal function. *Am J Med* 1979; 66:405–410.

27. Lewis EJ, Hunsicker LG, Bain RP, Rhode RD. The effect of angiotensin converting enzyme inhibition in diabetic nephropathy. *N Engl J Med* 1993; 323:1456–1462.

28. Epstein M. Calcium antagonists and renal protection. *Arch Intern Med* 1992; 152:1573–1584.

29. Levy D, Garrison RJ, Savage DD. Prognostic implications of echocardiographically determined left ventricular mass in the Framingham heart study. *N Engl J Med* 1990; 322:1561–1566.

30. Neill WA, Fluir-Lundeed JH. Myocardial oxygen supply in left ventricular hypertrophy and coronary heart disease. *Am J Cardiol* 1979; 44: 746–753.

31. Messerli FH, Soria F. Does a reduction in left ventricular hypertrophy reduce cardiovascular morbidity and mortality? *Drugs* 1992; 44:141–146.

32. Dahlöf B, Pennert K, Hansson L. Regression of left ventricular hypertrophy—a meta-analysis. *Clin Exp Hypertens* 1992; 14:173–180.

33. Messerli FH, Nuñez BD, Nuñez MM. Hypertension and sudden death: disparate effects of calcium entry blocker and diuretic therapy on cardiac dysrhythmias. *Arch Intern Med* 1989; 149:1263–1267.

34. Sen S, Tarazi RC, Bumpus FM. Cardiac hypertrophy and antihypertensive therapy. *Cardiovasc Res* 1977; 11:427–433.

35. Hoes AW, Grobbee DE, Lubsen J, et al. Diuretics, ß-blockers, and the risk for sudden cardiac death in hypertensive patients. *Ann Intern Med* 1995; 123:481–487.

36. Siscovick DS, Ragunathan TE, Psaty BM, et al. Diuretic therapy and the risk of primary cardiac arrest. *N Engl J Med* 1994; 330:1852–1857.

CHAPTER 15

Safety Issues in Combination Therapy, with Special Reference to Calcium Antagonists

Lionel H. Opie and Franz Messerli

Recently, there has been concern about the long-term safety of various antihypertensive drugs. For example, retrospective analyses of case-cohort studies suggest that both β-blockers and high-dose diuretics have been associated with sudden cardiac death. In the case of the calcium channel antagonists, although the "scare" has related to all agents, in reality the firm data relate high doses of short-acting nifedipine to increased mortality only in patients with acute ischemic syndromes or in elderly borderline hypertensives.

An important issue is whether any of these supposed dangers can be extrapolated to combination therapy. There are two major points to consider. First, how definite is the evidence for adverse effects of any class of drugs or for any specific drug? There, an important subquestion is whether and to what extent any proposed adverse effects are dose dependent and, if so, whether the "toxic" doses are those that are clinically used for hypertension therapy.

The second major issue is whether any of the antihypertensive combinations discussed in this book are likely to have additive, synergistic, or less-than-additive adverse effects. For example, if adverse effects are mediated by reflex adrenergic stimulation, then combination with a drug that has antiadrenergic properties such as a beta-blocker should, logically, improve safety.

EVIDENCE THAT QUESTIONS THE LONG-TERM SAFETY OF VARIOUS GROUPS OF ANTIHYPERTENSIVES

1. *Diuretics.* There have been several large outcome trials in which diuretics have been first-line drugs and these trials have shown beneficial effects. In none of them (not even in SHEP) was there a significant mortality reduction,

and in none was diuretic monotherapy the only permitted drug therapy (1). It is therefore not clear how much of the benefit of the therapy could be ascribed to diuretic therapy on its own and how much to the subsequently allowed combinations. Allowing for this limitation, it is encouraging to note that in the SHEP study, there was also a reduction in coronary heart disease (CHD) as an end point (1). When considered by the technique of meta-analysis, there are suggestions of a decreased total mortality and a decrease in coronary mortality, but the biggest and most consistent impact in all the trials has been in reduction of stroke (1). In the majority of studies the diuretic dose has been "high" (e.g., the MRC trial in the middle aged, bendrofluazide 10 mg) or "medium" (the MRC trial in the elderly, hydrochlorothiazide initial dose of 50 mg reduced to 25 mg; the EWPHE study, hydrochlothiazide 25 mg with potassium-retaining component). Only in the SHEP study in elderly hypertensives, was the dose "low" (chorthalidone 15 mg daily). Here the treatment sequence was a low-dose diuretic, medium dose (30 mg), and then combination with a beta-blocker, atenolol.

Within this framework there is evidence from a case-controlled study that high-dose diuretics (e.g., hydrochlorothiazide 100 mg) may be associated with arrhythmic cardiac deaths and that the harm can be lessened or removed by dose reduction or combining with a potassium-sparing component (2). Similar messages have come from another study in which the diuretic dose was not specifically looked at, but in which the patients were treated during an era in which high-dose diuretics were common (3). Thus, while the overall benefits of diuretic therapy for hypertension are not in doubt, two issues remain: (1) whether diuretic monotherapy can in fact achieve mortality reduction and (2) whether or not the doses of diuretic required to achieve control of hypertension by monotherapy could not have had adverse effects that would in turn lessen the theoretical benefit of blood pressure lowering, especially in relation to cardiac and hence overall mortality. These issues will probably never be answered, because there are no appropriate trials currently underway.

2. *β-Blockers.* Although β-blockers have been accorded privileged status, together with diuretics, as drugs of first choice for antihypertensive therapy in JNC-V, the actual number of β-blocker trials in which clear evidence of benefit was found are few. In the MRC trial in the middle aged, propranolol was only of benefit in reduction of coronary events in nonsmokers. The trial was underpowered for mortality, but there was not even a suggestion that mortality improved. In the MRC trial in the elderly, atenolol had no beneficial effects at all, but rather there was an adverse trend in mortality when compared with placebo. It is true that this trial has been severely criticized, especially for the high drop rate of about 25%. Furthermore, in both of the MRC trials, β-blockade monotherapy was only an initial option, and in case of no or imperfect response, the diuretic was added. In another trial, the STOP study in elderly Swedish hypertensives, initial β-blockade was again an option, but an

added diuretic was used in nearly two-thirds of the patients (See Chapter 13). In this study there were impressive reductions in cardiovascular and total mortality, but the benefits were not analyzed separately for β-blockers and diuretics.

Thus the existing data are insufficient to allow a judgment to be made about the effect of β-blockade, by itself, as an antihypertensive therapy that reduces mortality. Imperfect evidence suggests but does not prove a benefit for beta-blockade monotherapy on other end points such as stroke.

Against this background, the reported increase in sudden cardiac death or cardiac arrest in two retrospective case-control studies (2, 3) cannot be evaluated with certainty. The mechanism of this adverse effect is difficult to understand, but could perhaps speculatively be related to unopposed alpha-adrenergic activity or to overall sympathetic hyperactivity in periods of noncompliance during use of short-acting beta-blockers (4) or excess sinus node inhibition. It does remain possible that β-blockers have two opposing effects, namely a benefit by virtue of blood pressure reduction with a consequent reduction in hypertensive complications and therefore a trend to a reduced mortality, and conversely an adverse effect annulling at least some of the benefit otherwise found.

3. *Calcium antagonists.* Potential safety problems have caught the eye of many physicians, in part due to the large amount of publicity given in the popular press to the calcium blocker "scare." Most evidence focuses on the adverse effects of high doses of nifedipine in capsule form when inappropriately given, for example, to patients with acute ischemic syndromes (5, 6) or to elderly patients with trivial, borderline hypertension such as initial blood pressure readings of less than 160/90 mmHg (7).

It is likely that one mechanism for the adverse effects of short-acting calcium antagonists, especially the rapid vasodilators such as nifedipine that cause an acute tachycardia, is by reflex adrenergic and renin-angiotensin stimulation (8). Thus the combination of such an agent with a beta-blocker or an ACE inhibitor becomes logical. On the other hand, during chronic use, some calcium channel antagonists such as long acting verapamil (9), diltiazem, or amlodipine (4) tend to decrease rather than increase plasma catecholamine levels. Therefore it becomes necessary to consider the effects of the various calcium channel antagonists on plasma catecholamine levels.

4. *Alpha-adrenergic blockers.* In general, these compounds have a built-in safety factor in that they tend to decrease blood cholesterol levels. On the other hand, they are vasodilators and as such can be expected to activate the adrenergic and renin systems. In one case-control study, they increased the risk for AMI in patients with prior angina (10).

5. *ACE inhibitors.* Of all the classes of antihypertensive compounds, these appear to have the best safety record. They have been extensively tested at all stages of heart failure, and only when given intravenously to patients with early-phase AMI has there been adverse effects, presumably from excess hypotension (11). Of course, there are recognized side effects that may be lethal, such as angioedema or

renal failure, but these have not been sufficiently prominent to detract from the marked overall benefit in heart failure. Furthermore, there is indirect evidence that these agents have an indirect anti-ischemic effect and may reduce the risk of reinfarction or of unstable angina in patients with ischemic heart disease. Nonetheless, in the case of hypertension a word of caution is needed. There have been no outcome studies and the drug is clearly contraindicated in pregnancy hypertension.

6. *Angiotensin receptor blockers.* These, too, have no outcome studies in hypertension. A safety profile somewhat akin to that of the ACE inhibitors can be anticipated, with pregnancy hypertension and renal failure being absolute and relative contraindications. However, angioedema has only been reported very rarely and it is not clear that losartan was the culprit. This difference from the ACE inhibitors could be predicted because of the proposed role of bradykinin formation in angioedema.

7. *Conventional vasodilators.* This term is sometimes used to refer to old-style arteriolar vasodilators, such as hydralazine and minoxidil. In both cases there is indirect evidence for adrenergic-renin activation. For example, it was clinically well known that hydralazine, by promoting tachycardia, would aggravate angina, and that led to combination use of such agents with β-blockade. In the case of minoxidil, there is the combination of tachycardia with fluid retention, so that both a beta-blocker and a diuretic are required as cotreatment. Minoxidil also provokes left ventricular enlargement, supposedly by adrenergic activation. An interesting combination, well tested in a trial on heart failure (12), is that of hydralazine and a nitrate. It may be that the hydralazine lessened the tolerance otherwise expected with sustained nitrate therapy, so that added arteriolar (hydralazine) and venous dilatation (nitrates) could be obtained. This combination may be of practical importance in hypertensive patients with heart failure who are not responding to ACE inhibitors and diuretics.

8. *Centrally acting agents.* There are no large-scale outcome studies with agents such as methyldopa, clonidine, or their more modern counterparts (including those acting on imidazoline receptors). As these agents in general are indirect sympatholytics, it is reasonable to suppose that their safety profile would be adequate. But it must not be forgotten that methyldopa has a host of serious adverse side effects such as hepatitis, hemolytic anemia, and central depression. For most clinicians, these adverse possibilities far outweigh any benefit that might be accrued by an anti-sympathetic effect.

Only in the case of reserpine is there evidence from large trials of overall safety and benefit outweighing harm. A cancer scare, based on three separate retrospective case-control studies from three countries (13), lasted for some years but was eventually shown to be based on excessively small numbers and other statistical fallacies. As an adequate antihypertensive effect was achieved in several trials by low-dose reserpine, the only serious side effect, namely severe depression with suicide, was avoided. Thus, although this agent has gone out of popular use, it remains a safe and effective choice.

COMBINATIONS THAT MIGHT BENEFIT OR HARM

On existing knowledge, it might be anticipated that certain drug combinations would theoretically be beneficial in hypertension (Table 15-1) or harmful (Table 15-2). Such expectations guide the choice of combination drugs, especially in certain groups of patients such as diabetics. Conversely, certain combinations of drugs should be avoided, for example those causing excess vasodilation should be avoided in coronary heart disease. But such expectations do not deal with the fundamental issue of safety.

METHODS OF ADJUDGING SAFETY

There is no widely agreed definition of safety. What do we mean by a "safe" car? Safety is a balance between efficacy (the car gets you to the destination), efficiency (you get there sufficiently fast), and acceptable lack of unnecessary risk (the car does not overturn when going around a corner when driven at reasonable speed). The car is also free from unexpected defects (side effects) such as the doors flying open. Whatever defects there are in the car or dangers in the road, they may be overcome by a careful and experienced driver. Into the equation must also come cost—if the ideal safe car is so expensive that only a few can afford it, or if the car is a tank, then its use is not practical. The quality of life of pas-

TABLE 15-1. POTENTIALLY FATAL DOSE-RELATED SIDE EFFECTS OF ANTIHYPERTENSIVES[*]

Agent	High-Dose Effect	Reference
Reserpine	Suicide	(13)
Diuretics, non-potassium-sparing	Sudden cardiac arrest Diabetic ketosis	(2) (14)
Nifedipine, short acting	Death in UA or early AMI	(15)
	Death in nonhypertensive, very elderly patients	(7)

[*]Angioedema with ACE inhibitor is not dose related.
UA = unstable angina; AMI = acute myocardial infarction.

TABLE 15-2. ANTIHYPERTENSIVE DRUG COMBINATIONS THAT MAY THEORETICALLY BE BENEFICIAL

Combination	Reasons for Benefit
ß-blockers plus DHPs	Hemodynamic; less adrenergic effects
ß-blocker plus diuretic	Counters renin activation; less hypokalemia
CCAs plus ACE inhibitors	Counters renin activation; metabolically neutral (use in diabetics)
ACE inhibitor plus diuretic	Counters renin activation

DHP = dihydropyridine; CCA = calcium channel antagonist.

TABLE 15-3. ANTIHYPERTENSIVE DRUG COMBINATIONS THAT MAY THEORETICALLY BE HARMFUL

Combination	Reasons for Harm
ß-blockers (short acting?) plus high-dose diuretics	Added risk of sudden death
ß-blockers plus non-DHPs	Nodal and inotropic effects
CCAs plus vasodilators	Excess vasodilation
α-blockers plus vasodilators	Excess vasodilation

DHP = nondihydropyridine; CCA = calcium channel antagonist.

senger and driver must be good—it should be a pleasure to travel in the car. In brief, the car does its job at a reasonable cost with reasonable safety, depending on how it is driven, and gives pleasure to its occupants. The ideal "safe" drug is, likewise, not only efficacious, efficient, and free of unnecessary risk and unexpected side effects, but reasonable in price and gives a good quality of life. Such an ideal drug achieves its therapeutic aims without any adverse effects and with a good quality of life. But, coming back to the car analogy, a good driver (good doctor), by good judgment, can select the best route to take for a given car (drug selection) and drive at the best speed consistent with getting there (correct but not excess dosage). Adverse effects can be expected with any drug when used in too high a dose (driver goes too fast for the capacity of the car or the conditions of the road). Dose-related fatalities have been reported in relation to reserpine, diuretics, and short-acting nifedipine, all when used inappropriately (Tables 15-1 and 15-3).

QUALITY OF THE EVIDENCE ON SAFETY

At least five types of evidence can be adduced when considering safety (Table 15-4). The sources of data can be listed in an ascending hierarchy of significance: (1) reports of single cases or small series, (2) case-control studies, (3) cohort studies, (4) prospective randomized controlled trials (RCTs) that are properly randomized, and (5) well-conducted meta-analyses based on RCTs. Although, in general, the significance or the weight of the evidence provided goes up with each category of study, much depends on the details of the design. For example, a good cohort study can be better than a poorly designed randomized trial. Only in the case of meta-analysis are there definite criteria, laid down by Sacks and associates (22), and it seems as if many meta-analyses suffer from the defects of the trials on which they are based. One meta-analysis, by Furberg and colleagues (5), provided adverse information about the safety of short-acting nifedipine, yet contained so many errors that the conclusions have been doubted (6, 23).

In general, the grading of the significance of studies and the information about them still leaves much to be desired. Like the issue of safety, in the end subjective judgment seems inevitable, although the more experienced the judge, the more reliable the assessment. In this chapter the authors will attempt to give reasons for weighting a given study in

TABLE 15-4. Strengths and Defects of Various Types of Safety Studies

Type of Study and Example	Grading of Quality (scale 1–5)	Defects	Strong Points
Case reports	1	Unknown rate of adverse events	Helps drug choice in individual patient
Case control (16)	2	Entry criteria not solid (e.g., blood pressure data missing); cannot be randomized; drug choice bias may confound; no mortality data; retrospective; prospective trials with RCT results remain the gold standard	Serves as warning signal but is overridden by data from prospective studies
Cohort study (7, 17–20)	3	Nonrandomized; blood pressure data missing; no reason for drug selection; may confound; association not causation; changes in drugs used cannot be detected	Community based; simulates "real life"; can provide data on very old patients
Prospective, blinded RCT with major outcomes for CCAs: SPRINT I and II, DAVIT I and II, APSIS, TIBET	4–5	CCA trials only on ischemic heart disease; numbers underpowered to detect some rare side effects; may not be "real life" (e.g., very old often excluded); MRC trial: dropouts and crossovers; no outcome data for CCAs in hypertension	Provides solid data in clearly circumscribed population with valid criteria for entry and outcome clinical end points; reasonable evidence for safety of verapamil in anginal and post-AMI (21) populations, and in effort angina for slow-release nifedipine
Meta-analysis of several good RCTs	Potentially 5, mostly less (22)	Risk of grouping trials incorrectly	Can confirm major results; shows trends

RCT = randomized control trial; CCA = calcium channel antagonist; SPRINT = Secondary prevention reinfarction Israel nifedipine trial; DAVIT = Danish verapamil infarction trial; APSIS = angina prognosis study in Stockholm; TIBET = Total Ischaemic Burden European Trial; MRC = Medical Research Council.

a certain way, and this is particularly relevant in the case of evaluation of the safety of calcium channel antagonists.

ARE SHORT-ACTING CALCIUM CHANNEL BLOCKERS SAFE AS PART OF COMBINATION THERAPY FOR HYPERTENSION? LESSONS FROM VERAPAMIL AND NIFEDIPINE

Some of the problems in assessing drug safety can be illustrated by a current controversy in which the use of calcium blockers for hypertension has been questioned. The trigger has been a series of case-control and cohort studies in which it is claimed that short-acting calcium channel antagonists have various adverse effects, including an increase in myocardial infarction, increased total mortality, increased gastrointestinal hemorrhage (17), and most recently, the promotion of cancer in an aging population (17, 18).

In general, verapamil had no adverse effect on survival, whereas nifedipine did. One crucial factor distinguishing short-acting verapamil from the other two short-acting preparations is the existence of a unique pharmacological property, namely the prolongation of its half-life during chronic administration and the production of a long-acting metabolite, norverapamil (24) so that the short-acting form becomes longer acting. Thus, chronic therapy with verapamil, even its short-acting form, is not likely to be associated with major blood pressure swings nor with repetitive adrenergic activation. The results would be less risk of what Messerli (25) calls "bungee therapy." Furthermore, it would be easier to understand why a meta-analysis proposes that the short-acting non-dihydropyridines such as verapamil and diltiazem are more likely to induce regression of LVH than the short-acting dihydropyridines (8).

Safety of Short-Acting Verapamil in Ischemic Heart Disease

In ischemic heart disease, the case against calcium channel antagonists as a group rests on: (1) the meta-analysis of Furberg and colleagues (5), which suggested that excessive doses of short-acting nifedipine when used for indications for which it was not licensed, such as early-phase myocardial infarction, had a small increase in mortality provided that short- and not long-term follow-up was used; and (2) the case-control data of Psaty and associates (16), suggesting that there was an increased incidence of myocardial infarction in those treated for hypertension by short-acting nifedipine, verapamil, or diltiazem. In the first of these studies, verapamil was not mentioned and in the second, incidence of diabetes in the calcium antagonist group was about 50% higher than in the reference beta-blocker group. It was difficult to exclude the possibility that calcium antagonists, and in particular verapamil (26), had been selected preferentially for the diabetic group. Also, as pointed out by the authors, the higher doses of calcium antagonists that were associated with the increased incidence of myocardial infarction could have been a marker for more severe hypertension (no blood pressure levels are available in this case-control study). Finally, there was no increased mortality associated with the calcium antagonists, so that the supposed increase in AMI was in nonfatal infarcts. Yet it is precisely nonfatal infarcts that were lessened in a careful, prospective, blinded, randomized postmyocardial infarction trial, DAVIT II (27). Clearly data from such a prospective trial take precedence over those from a retrospective case-control study.

The safety of short-acting verapamil in ischemic heart disease is shown by the two DAVIT post-AMI studies, the second of which clearly shows that in patients not in heart failure at the onset, verapamil prevents reinfarction and the development of heart failure, combined with a trend toward reduced mortality (27). In another prospective, randomized, blinded study over 5 years on patients with effort angina, verapamil was as safe and as efficacious as the beta-blocker metoprolol, with similar fatality rates and no trend toward increased AMI (28). The total number of patients given verapamil in these three trials was 1,952.

Safety of Verapamil and Diltiazem in Meta-Analyses of Postinfarct Populations

In three meta-analyses, diltiazem and verapamil have been considered together on the basis that both reduce heart rate and both have been studied in placebo-controlled trials in similar postinfarct populations. In 936 patients recovering from non-Q infarcts (29), there was a 35% reduction in cardiac death or nonfatal reinfarction over 12 to 18 months. Taking together all the 5,677 patients from three trials over a mean follow-up time of 550 days (30–32), Boden and colleagues (33) found a reduction in cardiac death plus reinfarction of 12% (CI, 0.77–0.99). Messerli (25), reporting on the same three studies, found that the benefit obtained by verapamil or diltiazem could be localized to those with hypertension, with a risk ratio of 0.76 (CI, 0.61–0.95). In none of these three meta-analyses, however, was there any reduction in total mortality.

The general picture that emerges is that when these drugs are correctly used, they are safe and have benefits. This finding is in contrast to that of Koenig and associates (19), who found in a cohort study that short-acting diltiazem had adverse effects with a risk ratio for mortality of 1.55 (CI, 1.04–2.32) in a postinfarct population. This observation, however, is not placebo controlled and it seems that the majority of patients in the diltiazem group were in heart failure, as judged by the use of diuretics (54%) and ACE inhibitors (10%). It is already established from the MDPIT trial that diltiazem increases the mortality in postinfarct patients with heart failure.

Safety of Short-Acting Nifedipine and Diltiazem: the Israeli Study

In a very large cohort study (20) on 11,575 patients with coronary artery disease who had been considered but not entered for a trial with bezafibrate, mortality data were obtained after a mean follow-up of 3.2 years. The nifedipine used in

1,999 patients was predominantly of the short-acting variety in doses of 30 to 60 mg/day. The diltiazem used in 3,320 patients was not stipulated. These agents did not increase mortality. Rather, there was a trend toward decreased mortality as the severity of the angina increased. This study suggests that even the short-acting agents, when properly used with due care, do not have any increase in total mortality.

Safety of Short-Acting Verapamil in Elderly Cohort Studies

In two of the elderly cohort studies, verapamil was no different from beta-blockers. For example, in the elderly survival study, in which patients with hypertension were diagnosed by a variety of means including "self-diagnosis," the mortality rate with verapamil was indistinguishable from that with beta-blockers (7). In the cancer study, the incidence of fatal cancer with verapamil was 7.8 (CI, 0.25–3.29, ns) versus 7.1 in beta-blockers. It needs to be emphasized that the numbers in this study are so small (N = 2 for verapamil) that the data relating to fatal cancers are not valid. The incidence of non-fatal cancer in those in the verapamil group was increased, but again the numbers were small (N = 10 for verapamil). Regarding the increase in nonfatal cancer reported for all calcium channel antagonists (17), the overall risk ratio was between 1.42 (unadjusted data) and 1.72 (adjusted data). Diltiazem was without risk. These risks should be compared with the relative risk of 1.8 to 2.2 for renal cell carcinoma for diuretic use (34), and with the numerous nonspecific factors that increase the risk of cancer by similar factors (35).

It must also be considered that there were only 451 users of calcium channel antagonists in the Pahor study (17). These are really small numbers when compared with approximately 1,000 patients given atenolol in the prospective MRC study (36). Atenolol was associated with a death rate from cancer of 15.8 per 1,000 patient-years, whereas in the much smaller nonrandomized Pahor study (18) a very similar death rate was associated with calcium antagonists as a group. It took a retrospective cohort study on 6,528 patients to disprove the link between atenolol and cancer and to call it a "chance finding" (37). The latter authors point out that "the number of events in a study determines the statistical power." There were only 27 events in the first Pahor study and 47 in the second. Thus, at the very least, the data in the Pahor studies need to be interpreted with considerable reserve. It should also be recalled that reserpine was once thought to have breast cancer as a side effect, as a result of no less than three epidemiological studies, and a warning editorial in *Lancet*, yet this risk was subsequently disproved almost 10 years later, when many more patients were analyzed.

Gastrointestinal Bleeding in the Elderly: A New Side Effect of Verapamil?

In all of these studies, verapamil has been the major culprit only in the case of gastrointestinal bleeds in a population with an arbitrary age cutoff point of 67 years, with an increased relative risk of 2.3 (17). This finding accords with the known vasodilating and antiplatelet effects of verapamil, the latter providing a mechanism for the reduction of reinfarction. *Clearly, suspected gastrointestinal bleeds or bleeding points become a contraindication to verapamil in this age group.* How serious the risk is must be judged in relation to the estimate that 86 patients must be treated for 1 year to produce one additional gastrointestinal bleed (38).

CATECHOLAMINE STIMULATION AND DIVERSE ADVERSE EFFECTS OF SHORT-ACTING CALCIUM CHANNEL ANTAGONISTS (NIFEDIPINE VS. VERAPAMIL)

In general, the major culprit has been short-acting nifedipine (capsule form). This is the agent with the worst mortality in the cohort study of Pahor and colleagues, and the highest risk of fatal cancer in the other Pahor study (relative risk for fatal cancer with nifedipine [3.74; CI, 1.30–10.78]). This is also the preparation that when used in high doses has had adverse effects in patients with acute ischemic syndromes, as in the Muller study (15) and in the second SPRINT study (39). It is the only agent considered in the meta-analysis of Furberg and associates (5). Why is there this striking difference from short-acting verapamil? For example, in the Pahor survival study, the relative risk for nifedipine versus verapamil was 2.6 (CI, 1.3–5.4) and the authors emphasize that it is important to realize that the nifedipine was of the short-acting variety.

A possible explanation for the adverse effects of this preparation of nifedipine in the setting of acute ischemia is the reflex adrenergic stimulation that is clinically manifest as a tachycardia, with an enhancement rather than the desired decrease of the myocardial oxygen consumption. That this explanation is correct is supported by the finding in two studies on unstable angina or threatened infarction, in which the addition of a beta-blockade gave an improved result (15, 40).

Can the higher rates of cancer also be linked to the short duration of action of nifedipine, the intermittent high blood levels, and vigorous intermittent sympathetic stimulation? The hypothesis recently proposed is that all calcium antagonists inhibit the antineoplastic process of apoptosis and therefore may promote cancer (18). An *alternate hypothesis* is that excess adrenergic stimulation could enhance the activity of the signal pathway that links the $alpha_1$-receptor to the messengers that also respond to the mitogenic agents, the phorbol esters (41). Thus, agents giving less sympathetic stimulation would be less mitogenic, thereby explaining the differences between nifedipine and verapamil in relation to fatal cancer. This mechanism receives support from the links between tachycardia and prostatic cancer (42).

An important finding is that short-acting verapamil provokes less rise of plasma noradrenaline than does short-acting nifedipine for a similar fall of blood pressure (43). In the case of short-acting verapamil, a total daily dose of 240 mg given for several months did not increase plasma noradrenaline whereas a dose of 480 mg daily did (43). These differences are of interest because long-acting preparations in a dose of 240 to 480 mg daily *decreased* plasma noradrenaline (9, 44) and blunted the pressor response to cardiovascular stress (45). Of interest, the dose of 240 mg of the short-acting preparation was regarded as the modal daily dose by Psaty and colleagues (16), and it was a higher dose that might have had adverse effects in increasing the incidence of non-fatal AMI. Conversely, in the prospective post-AMI study (32), the daily dose of verapamil that decreased reinfarction was 160 mg three times daily (total dose, 480 mg).

Because prospective randomized studies provide data of a higher hierarchy and greater validity than do case-control studies, two conclusions can be made. First, short-acting verapamil even when given in a dose of 480 mg daily, which is likely to give a modest increase in plasma catecholamines, has beneficial effects, such as platelet inhibition, that outweigh any catechol-induced harm. Therefore, not surprisingly, in the survival cohort study (7) not even higher doses of verapamil had harmful effects when compared with a beta-blocker. Secondly, long-acting verapamil, known to lower blood catecholamine levels, might have given a better result in the DAVIT studies than the short-acting preparation.

IMPLICATIONS FOR THE SAFETY OF LONG-ACTING CALCIUM BLOCKERS

If the basic hypothesis can be made that part of the benefits of verapamil reside in its potentially low catecholamine profile, then certain conclusions can be made. First, to avoid adrenergic activation would require either long-acting preparations, or the combination of short-acting nifedipine with a beta-blocker, or the use of short-acting verapamil. It needs to be emphasized that it is evidently wrong to lump the short-acting calcium channel antagonists together. The "scare stories" largely relate to short-acting nifedipine, with short-acting verapamil relatively free of problems, and with short-acting diltiazem somewhere in between (7). Nonetheless, the temptation to "outlaw" completely short-acting nifedipine must be avoided. The blood pressure-lowering effects of this drug can outweigh even vigorous adrenergic stimulation, at least in the case of silent ischemia (46). From the safety point of view, its use in severe, urgent hypertension has not been properly evaluated, although there are known risks such as the precipitation of ischemia or infarction (21). Possibly the lives of many patients with severe coronary spasm have been saved by the use of short-acting nifedipine.

In the case of truly long-acting compounds there is evidence that plasma catecholamine levels are decreased (4), so that by inference they should be safe in patients with stable coronary artery disease (8). Furthermore, they should and do achieve regression of LVH (4). In contrast, with twice-daily felodipine, even when the latter is given with concurrent beta-blocker therapy, there is no regression of LVH (4).

There is, however, no evidence as yet for the safety of long-acting dihydropyridines in acute ischemic syndromes.

Much still remains to be learned about the degree of adrenergic activation that can be found in patients on long-acting dihydropyridine-type calcium channel antagonists. For example, plasma catecholamines fell modestly (10% to 20%) with amlodipine over 6 months (4), whereas even with extended-release felodipine, there was no change in plasma catecholamine levels over 1 month (9) or, in another study (47), increased levels after 2 months of treatment. Such changes in catecholamine patterns can be linked to the extent of regression of LVH (4, 8), and although inferential intuitive evidence is that a low catecholamine profile will give verapamillike benefit to patients with ischemic heart disease, the hard data must still be obtained. It is, for example, known that intensely stressful situations can still evoke adrenergic activation in patients treated even by the very long-acting dihydropyridine amlodipine (45), which argues for combination therapy of long-acting dihydropyridines with a beta-blocker for patients with prominent risk of unstable angina or AMI.

At present there is a large number of studies in progress regarding various calcium channel antagonists in hypertension, involving no less than 74,032 patients. When these studies are available, it is likely that calcium channel antagonists will be among the best-researched compounds in the management of hypertension. It is also likely that these studies will remove any lingering doubts about long-term safety, when appropriately used for correct indications in the correct doses.

When diuretics do not work, or are contraindicated or not tolerated, there is no compelling reason to choose beta-blockers rather than calcium antagonists as second-line therapy (48). When calcium antagonists are chosen, and cost considerations are important (for example, in third-world countries), then generic verapamil, nominally short-acting but in reality longer acting, becomes a reasonable choice with due regard for established cardiac contraindications such as heart block or systolic heart failure. In general, however, most clinicians are going to opt for one of the long-acting calcium channel antagonists as their choice for antihypertensive therapy.

PROPOSALS AND CONCLUSIONS

1. Data on safety of drugs come from a variety of sources that have varying values depending on the method of data collection. In general, case-control and cohort studies carry less weight than randomized, controlled, prospective trials. In addition, in the case of a meta-analysis, the subjective interpretations of the observers can be crucial. For example, can the various studies really be combined? Several of the recently reported adverse effects of various antihypertensives, including high-dose diuretics, beta-blockers, and calcium antagonists, have stemmed from nonrandomized studies that are open to criticism.

2. Only in a few cases has combination therapy been assessed from the safety point of view. One good example is

the evidence collected only from case-control studies, but nonetheless regarded as valid by the present authors, that the combination of a diuretic with a potassium-sparing agent confers mortality benefit when compared with high doses of a diuretic alone. Such data by extrapolation favor but do not prove the safety of the combination of a diuretic with an ACE inhibitor. There are also rather imperfect data suggesting that the addition of a beta-blocker to a nonpotassium-sparing diuretic is safer than a nonpotassium-sparing diuretic alone (3). Furthermore, the trials on the elderly reviewed in Chapter 1 provide indirect evidence that the combination of a beta-blocker and a low-dose diuretic is not only safe but efficacious, at least in the elderly.

3. In the only case-control study that has reported on the risk of myocardial infarction in hypertensive patients treated by combination therapy, there was no increased risk of calcium channel antagonist combined with diuretic compared with beta-blocker or ACE inhibitor plus diuretic, but the numbers were small and a real effect could easily have been missed (49).

4. In the elderly cohort study of Pahor and colleagues (7), the survival with verapamil was almost identical to that found with β-blockade. The survival with ACE inhibitors was, if anything, slightly better. Thus, except for some unexpected adverse interaction, the safety of the combination of verapramil and an ACE inhibitor should be acceptable.

5. A consideration of the basic properties of the various agents is also of importance in the absence of firm outcome data for combination therapy. For example, the adverse effects of short-acting nifedipine may involve reflex adrenergic stimulation, which can be countered by the addition of a beta-blocker. Alternatively, an agent such as verapamil, which in itself does not increase but rather decreases blood catecholamine levels, may be preferred. Nonetheless it is noted that verapamil does have negative inotropic effects that have led to exclusion of postinfarct patients with heart failure from the DAVIT II trial (32). Logically, a combination with an ACE inhibitor may be considered safer. Trials on this point are currently underway (50).

6. Regarding the combination of a calcium channel antagonist with a beta-blocker, the established clinical adage that the dihydropyridines combine better because of their absence of nodal effects and lesser negative inotropic qualities still holds. Nonetheless, with clinical attention to additive nodal and negative inotropic effects, nondihydropyridines can also be successfully combined with beta-blockers.

References

1. Thijs L, Fagard R, Lijnen P, et al. A meta-analysis of outcome trials in elderly hypertensives. *J Hypertens* 1992; 10:1103–1109.

2. Siscovick DS, Raghunathun TE, Psaty BM. Diuretic therapy for hypertension and the risk of primary cardiac arrest. *N Engl J Med* 1994; 330:1852–1857.

3. Hoes AW, Grobbee DE, Lubsen J, et al. Diuretics, β-blockers, and the risk for sudden cardiac death in hypertensive patients. *Ann Intern Med* 1995; 123:481–487.

4. Leenen FH. l,4-dihydropyridines versus beta-blockers for hypertension: Are either safe for the heart? *Cardiovasc Drugs Ther* 1996; 10:397–402.

5. Furberg CD, Psaty BM, Meyer JV. Nifedipine dose-related increase in mortality in patients with coronary heart disease. *Circulation* 1995; 92:1326–1331.

6. Opie LH, Messerli FH. Nifedipine and mortality. Grave defects in the dossier. *Circulation* 1995; 92:1068–1073.

7. Pahor M, Guralnik JM, Corti M, et al. Long term survival and use of antihypertensive medications in older persons. *J Am Geriatr Soc* 1995; 43:1191–1197.

8. Ruzicka M, Leenen FH. Relevance of 24 h blood pressure profile and sympathetic activity for outcome on short-versus long-acting 1,4-dihydropyridines. *Am J Hypertens* 1996; 9:86–94.

9. Kailasam MT, Parmer RJ, Cervenka JH, et al. Divergent effects of dihydropyridine and phenylalkylamine calcium channel antagonist classes on autonomic function in human hypertension. *Hypertension* 1995; 26:143–149.

10. Aursnes I, Litleskare I, Froyland H, Abdelnoor M. Association between various drugs used for hypertension and risk of acute myocardial infarction. *Blood Press* 1995; 4:157–163.

11. CONSENSUS II, Swedberg K, Held P, et al. Effects of the early administration of enalapril on mortality in patients with acute myocardial infarction. Results of the Co-operative Scandinavian Enalapril Survival Study II (CONSENSUS II). *N Engl J Med* 1992; 327:678–684.

12. Cohn JN, Archibald DG, Ziesche S. Effect of vasodilator therapy on mortality in chronic congestive heart failure. Results of Veterans Administration Cooperative Study. *N Engl J Med* 1986; 314; 1547–1552.

13. Anonymous. Rauwolfia derivatives and cancer. *Lancet* 1974; 2:701–702.

14. Cranston WI, Juel-Jensen BE, Semmence AM, et al. Effects of oral diuretics on raised arterial pressure. *Lancet* 1963; 2:966–969.

15. Muller JE, Turi ZG, Pearl DL, et al. Nifedipine and conventional therapy for unstable angina pectoris: a randomized, double-blind comparison. *Circulation* 1984; 69:728–739.

16. Psaty BM, Heckbert SR, Koepsell TD, et al. The risk of myocardial infarction associated with antihypertensive drug therapies. *JAMA* 1995; 274:620–625.

17. Pahor M, Furalnik JM, Furberg CD, et al. Risk of gastrointestinal haemorrhage with calcium antagonists in hypertensive persons over 67 years old. *Lancet* 1996; 347:1061–1065.

18. Pahor M, Guralnik JM, Salive ME, et al. Do calcium channel blockers increase the risk of cancer? *Am J Hypertens* 1996; 9:695–699.

19. Koenig W, Lowel H, Lewis M, Hormann M. Long-term survival after myocardial infarction: relationship with thrombolysis and discharge medication. Results of the Augsburg myocardial infarction follow-up study. *Eur Heat J* 1996; 17:1199–1206.

20. Braun S, Boyko V, Behar S, et al. Calcium antagonists and mortality in patients with coronary artery disease: a cohort study of 11,575 patients. *J Am Coll Cardiol* 1996; 28:7–11.

21. O'Mailia J, Sander GE, Giles TD. Nifedipine-associated myocardial ischemia or infarction in the treatment of hypertensive urgencies. *Ann Intern Med* 1987; 107:185–186.

22. Sacks HJ, Berrier J, Reitman D, et al. Meta-analyses of randomized controlled trials. *N Engl J Med* 1987; 316:450–455.

23. Rafflenbeul W. Nifedipine in acute coronary syndromes: Furberg's refrain revisted. *Eur Heart J* 1996; 17:1147–1152.

24. Schwartz JB, Keefe DL, Kirsten E, et al. Prolongation of verapamil elimination kinetics during chronic oral administration. *Am Heart J* 1982; 104:198–203.

25. Messerli F. Whatever happened to the calcium antagonist controversy? [editorial]. *JACC* 1996; 28:12–13.

26. Rojdmark S, Andersson DEH. Influence of verapamil on human glucose tolerance. *Am J Cardiol* 1986; 57:39D–43D.

27. Fischer Hansen J. The Danish Study Group on Verapamil in Myocardial Infarction. Treatment with verapamil during and after an acute myocardial infarction: a review based on the Danish verapamil infarction trials I and II. *J Cardiovasc Pharmacol* 1991; 18(Suppl 6):S20–S25.

28. Rehnqvist N, Hjemdahl P, et al. The angina prognosis study in Stockholm (APSIS). Effects of metoprolol vs verapamil in patients with stable angina pectoris. *Eur Heart J* 1996; 17:76–81.

29. Boden WE, Fischer Hansen J, Lau J, Roberts R. Beneficial effect of heart rate-lowering calcium channel blockers (diltiazem, verapamil) on reducing long-term (12–18 month) cardiac death and nonfatal reinfarction in patients recovering from acute non-Q-wave myocardial infarction [abstract]. *Circulation* 1995; 92(Suppl I):I-81.

30. Multicenter Diltiazem Postinfarction Trial Research Group. The effect of diltiazem on mortality and reinfarction after myocardial infarction. *N Engl J Med* 1983; 391:385–392.

31. Danish Study Group on Verapamil in Myocardial Infarction. Verapamil in acute myocardial infarction. *Br J Clin Pharmacol* 1986; 21:197S–204S.

32. Danish Study Group of Verapamil in Myocardial Infarction. The effects of verapamil on mortality and major events after myocardial infarction. The Danish Verapamil Infarction Trial II (DAVIT II). *Am J Cardiol* 1990; 66:779–785.

33. Boden W, Messerli FH, Fisher Hansen J, Schectman KB. Heart rate-lowering calcium channel blockers (diltiazem, verapamil) do not adversely affect long-term cardiac death or non-fatal infarction in post-infarction patients: data pooled from 3 randomized, placebo-controlled clinical trials of 5,677 patients. *Am J Cardiol* 1996; 27:319A.

34. Weinmann S, Glass AG, Weiss NS, et al. Use of diuretics and other antihypertensive medications in relation to the risk of renal cell cancer. *Am J Epidemiol* 1994; 140:792–804.

35. Taubes G. Epidemiology faces its limits. *Science* 1995; 269:164–169.

36. Medical Research Council trial of treatment of hypertension in older adults: principal results. *BMJ* 1992; 304:405–412.

37. Hole DJ, Hawthorne VM, McGhee SM, et al. Incidence of mortality from cancer in hypertensive patients. *Br Med J* 1993; 306:609–611.

38. Gordon RD. Calcium antagonists and gastrointestinal haemorrhage: the balancing act. *Lancet* 1996; 347:1056.

39. SPRINT II, Goldbourt U, Behar S, et al. Early administration of nifedipine in suspected acute myocardial infarction. The Secondary Prevention Reinfarction Israel Nifedipine Trial 2 Study. *Arch Intern Med* 1993; 153:345–353.

40. HINT Trial Holland Interuniversity Nifedipine/Metoprolol. Early treatment of unstable angina in the coronary care unit; a randomised, double-blind, placebo controlled comparison of recurrent ischaemia in patients treated with nifedipine or metoprolol or both. *Br Heart J* 1986; 56:400–413.

41. Opie LH. Calcium channel blockers for hypertension—dissecting the evidence for adverse effects. *Am J Hypertens* 1997; (in press).

42. Gann PH, Daviglus ML, Dyer AR, Stamler J. Heart rate and prostate cancer mortality. Results of a prospective analysis. *Cancer Epidemiol* 1995; 4:611–616.

43. Agabiti-Rosei E, Muiesan ML, Romanelli G, et al. Similarities and differences in the antihypertensive effect of two calcium antagonist drugs, verapamil and nifedipine. *J Am Coll Cardiol* 1986; 7:916–924.

44. Wallen NH, Held C, Rehnqvist N, Hjemdahl P. Platelet aggregability in vivo is attenuated by verapamil but not by metroprolol in patients with stable angina pectoris. *Am J Cardiol* 1995; 75:1–6.

45. Nazzaro P, Manzari M, Merlo R, et al. Antihypertensive treatment with verapamil and amlodipine. *Eur Heart J* 1995; 92:1227–1284.

46. Lee JA, Allen DG. Changes in intracellular free calcium concentration during long exposures to simulated ischemia in isolated mammalian ventricular muscle. *Circ Res* 1992; 71:58–69.

47. Lindqvist M, Kahan T, Melcher A, Hjemdahl P. Acute and chronic calcium antagonist treatment elevates sympathetic activity in primary hypertension. *Hypertension* 1994; 24:287–296.

48. Opie LH. Calcium channel antagonists should be among the first-line drugs in the management of cardiovascular disease. *Cardiovasc Drugs Ther* 1996; 10:455–458.

49. Jick H, Derby LE, Gurewich V, Vasilakis K. The risk of myocardial infarction associated with antihypertensive drug treatment in persons with uncomplicated essential hypertension. *Pharmacotherapy* 1996; 16:321–326.

50. Fischer Hansen J, Tingsted L, Rasmussen V, et al. Verapamil and angiotensin-converting enzyme inhibitors in patients with coronary artery disease and reduced left ventricular ejection fraction. *Am J Cardiol* 1996; 77:(in press).